OECD Health Policy Studies

Better Ways to Pay for Health Care

Divya Srivastava,
Michael Mueller,
Emily Hewlett

OECD
BETTER POLICIES FOR BETTER LIVES

Please cite this publication as:
OECD (2016), *Better Ways to Pay for Health Care*, OECD Health Policy Studies, OECD Publishing, Paris.
http://dx.doi.org/10.1787/9789264258211-en

ISBN 978-92-64-25820-4 (print)
ISBN 978-92-64-25821-1 (PDF)

Series: OECD Health Policy Studies
ISSN 2074-3181 (print)
ISSN 2074-319X (online)

The statistical data for Israel are supplied by and under the responsibility of the relevant Israeli authorities. The use of such data by the OECD is without prejudice to the status of the Golan Heights, East Jerusalem and Israeli settlements in the West Bank under the terms of international law.

Photo credits: Cover © Alexander Lukin/Shutterstock.com; © iStockphoto.com/-WaD-; © iStockphoto.com/Amornism; Oleg Bobrek/Thinkstock; © vladis.studio/Shutterstock.com

Corrigenda to OECD publications may be found on line at: *www.oecd.org/about/publishing/corrigenda.htm*.

Foreword

In nearly all industries, payments for services or products reflect short-term performance or long-term value. Yet in health care, most payments to health providers have done neither. Instead, they have often simply rewarded greater volume of services whether needed or not. Recently, attention has moved away from rewarding volume of health care to quality and efficiency. Changing epidemiology and care models for an ageing population, managing of patients with complex health needs and scarce resources, all make it imperative to change how we pay for health services.

This new publication considers payment innovations in OECD countries. These include different new models: "add-on payments", including pay-for-performance, whereby health care providers are rewarded for delivering more co-ordinated, safer and effective care; "bundled payments", whereby payments for all services provided to a patient with a medical problem are pooled together; and "population-based payments", whereby the payment covers most care needs of patients. The analysis shows that all three payment innovations show promise. Many patients are starting to experience improved quality care and improved health outcomes as a result. Add-on payments that reward providers for their efforts to better co-ordinate health care for a patient have shown their potential to improve quality, while controlling costs. Pay-for-performance schemes have improved care processes although they have not delivered a breakthrough in outcomes and quality of care. A number of bundled payments have raised the experience and effectiveness of care for patients, and generated cost savings. Population-based payments have helped overcome fragmentation of care, in the majority of cases leading to both better outcomes and a slowdown in health spending growth.

Policy makers should scale up these positive results by implementing these payment reforms more broadly in their health systems. This is not always easy, of course. The design of payment innovations requires careful setting of rewards and tariffs based on evidence, as well as strong investment in IT capability by both providers and payers. Stakeholders need to be brought on-board and involved throughout the process. A sometimes difficult balance must be struck between the need to generate new data and evidence on which to calibrate payments, and added administrative burden. And a culture of more systematic and independent evaluation of impact must become more common practice.

Despite these difficulties, this publication has shown that investment in payment innovations generate good bang for the buck. Fundamentally, they are helping to align payers and providers, and more broadly health systems, towards what they should aim for – that is, best outcomes for patients given resources invested. Scaled up, these payment innovations will bring about system-wide effects, including a stronger focus on what patients need the most and greater generation of data to feed decision-making processes. Policy makers should not delay any further implementing innovations such as those presented in this report. The path towards a health care system where providers are rewarded for what they are able to deliver to patients – not simply what they can do – has already been very long. Now, it is the time to shorten it.

ACKNOWLEDGEMENTS

The OECD project on payment systems was managed by Divya Srivastava. This book was edited by Divya Srivastava, Michael Mueller and Emily Hewlett. The chapters were written by Michael Mueller (Chapters 1, 2 and 4), Divya Srivastava (Chapters 1 and 3) and Emily Hewlett (Chapters 1 and 2).

We would like to thank the authors and experts who drafted sections of the publication or provided detailed information on their countries and without whom this book would not have been possible: Ricarda Milstein (Universität Hamburg) and Carl Rudolf Blankart (Universität Hamburg) on innovations in Germany in Chapters 2 and 4; Benjamin Gershlick (Health Foundation) and John Henderson (Department of Health) on innovations in the United Kingdom in Chapter 3; Gioia Buckley and Arthur Sweetman (McMaster University) on innovations in Ontario, Canada in Chapter 2; Shuli Brammli-Greenberg (University of Haifa); Ruth Waitzberg (Smokler Center for Health Policy Research at Myers-JDC-Brookdale Institute); Vadim Perman (Ministry of Health); Ronni Gamzu (Tel Aviv Medical Center) on innovations in Israel in Chapter 1; Chun Yee Wong, Chinzhou Mu, Jane Hall and Kees van Gool (University of Technology Sydney) for information on diabetes in Australia in Chapter 2; Grégoire de Lagasnerie and Anne-Sophie Aguadé (Caisse nationale de l'assurance maladie des travailleurs salariés) for information on diabetes in France in Chapter 2; Floris. P. Vlaanderen (Radboud University Medical Center and ParkinsonNet), Marjan J. Faber (ParkinsonNet and Radboud University Medical Center), Marten Munneke (ParkinsonNet), Bastiaan R. Bloem (ParkinsonNet, Nijmegen Centre for Evidence-Based Practice, Radboud University Medical Center) and Patrick P.T. Jeurissen (Radboud University Medical Center and Ministry of Health Welfare and Sport) on innovations in the Netherlands in Chapter 3; Jeroen Struijs (National Institute for Public Health and the Environment) for information on diabetes in the Netherlands in Chapter 3; Adolfo Martínez Valle (Ministry of Health) and Miguel A. González Block (Universidad Anáhuac) on innovations in Mexico in Chapter 2; Camilla Beck Olsen and Geir Brandborg (Ministry of Health) on innovations in Norway in Chapter 2. Alexandre Lourenço (Nova Healthcare Initiative – Nova School of Business and Economics and Coimbra Hospital and University Centre) on innovations in Portugal in Chapters 2 and 3.

We would also like to thank the national and international experts who provided valuable comments to the project and country examples: Cheryl Cashin (Results for Development Institute); Jonas Wohlin (Ivbar Institute, Sweden). We thank those who attended the experts' meeting held in Paris on 7-8 April 2014, and officials from the Health Ministries who provided helpful comments to the country examples and to those who attended the OECD Health Committee meetings held in Paris on 25-26 June 2015.

We received invaluable support and guidance from Valérie Paris throughout the course of the project. We are extremely grateful to Agnès Couffinhal, Francesca Colombo and Mark Pearson for their comments on earlier drafts. We thank Judy Zinneman, Isabelle Vallard and Anna Irvin-Sigal for the editorial and administrative support during the course of the project, Daphné Guilmard (former OECD intern) for research, and Marlène Mohier in the final stages of the preparation of the manuscript.

Table of contents

Figures

Tables

Acronyms and abbreviations

ACE	Acute care episode
ACES	Regional primary care organisations
ACO	Accountable Care Organisations
ALD	Long-term conditions (*Affections de longue durée*)
AMT	Abbreviated Mental Test
ARB	Angiotensin II receptor blocker
ARS	Regional health agencies (*Agences régionales de santé*)
BMI	Body mass index
BPT	Best Practice Tariff
BVA	Federal Insurance Agency
CABG	Coronary artery bypass graft surgery
CAD	Coronary artery disease
CAPI	Contract to improve individual practices (*Contrat d'amélioration des pratiques individuelles*)
CMS	Centres for Medicare and Medicaid Services
CNAMTS	French Health Insurance Fund (*Caisse nationale de l'assurance maladie des travailleurs salariés*)
COPD	Chronic obstructive pulmonary disease
DMP	Disease Management Program
DRG	Diagnosis-related group
EHR	Electronic Health Record
ENMR	Experimentation of new modes of remuneration (*Expérimentations de nouveaux modes de rémunération*)
FFS	Fee-for-service
FHU	Family Health Unit
GP	General practitioner
HAS	Haute Autorité de Santé
HRG	Healthcare Resource Group
HSC	Health Systems Characteristics Survey

ICHOM	International Consortium for Health Outcomes Measurement
IHA	Integrated Healthcare Association
IVD	In vitro diagnostic
KCPS	Korean Case Payment System
K-DRG	Korean diagnosis related group
LTC	Long-term care
LVSD	Left Ventricular Systolic Dysfunction
MEPS	Medical Expenditure Panel Survey
NHS	National Health Service
NICE	National Institute for Health and Clinical Excellence
P4P	Pay-for-performance
PCP	Pneumocystis carinii pneumonia
PGP	Physician Group Practice
PIP	Practice Incentive Program
PN	ParkinsonNet
PPP	Public private partnership
PRG	Procedure related group
QBF	Quality Based Financing
QOF	Quality and Outcomes Framework
RACGP	Royal Australian College of General Practitioners
RHA	Regional Health Authority
ROSP	Remuneration of public health objectives (*Rémunération sur objectifs de santé publique*)
SIP	Service incentive payment
UHI	Universal health insurance

Executive summary

How health care providers are paid is one of the key policy levers that countries have to drive health system performance. However, health providers are still paid in traditional ways – through fee-for-service (FFS), capitation, salary, global budgets or more recently diagnosis-related groups (DRGs). These give incentives for undesirable behaviours, for instance over-provision of services or inattention to clinical needs. More should be done to align payer and provider incentives so that payment is based on delivering value to patients.

Countries are stepping up to meet this challenge. Many healthcare providers in OECD countries are successfully delivering greater quality care thanks to innovative reforms to the way in which they are paid. In addition to making better use of traditional payment systems, OECD countries have been experimenting with new ways of paying providers to improve co-ordination, quality, outcomes and efficiency of care. Experiences of 12 countries shows three broad recent trends in payment innovations:

- Add-on payments paid on top of existing payment methods, which are tied to specific expectations of the care provider. Such payments are being used to encourage co-ordination, improve care quality and reward performance.
- Bundled payments for episodes of care or for chronic conditions, which aim to improve care quality and reduce costs.
- Population-based payments in which groups of health providers receive payments on the basis of the population covered, in order to provide most healthcare services for that population, with built-in quality and cost-containment requirements.

These innovative approaches to pay health providers have been successful in improving some aspects of the quality of care, health outcomes and/or reducing the costs of care provision. For example, add-on payments are used in different domains of care – payments for co-ordination are relatively easy to implement while payments to reward achievement are more complex. Bundled payments have improved protocols of care, however tariff setting is more complex and brings an added administrative burden. Population-based payments show slower health spending growth but whether they can contribute to make health systems more performing in the long-run will remain to be seen.

The three different types of innovations examined in this report differ in their complexity and some of them give providers more financial flexibility and autonomy in organising care for their patients. A common feature is that providers have been increasingly willing to accept payment models that entail more financial risk for them, and payers have been more actively engaged in shaping modes of payment in countries where they are allowed to play a more strategic role.

Experience over the last decades has shown that payment systems evolve constantly and providers adapt behaviours over time so that the effectiveness of the incentives declines over time. But even if innovative payments have not systematically proven yet that they add value, they can have positive system-wide effects by inducing better data collection, clarifying health policy objectives and leading to a more informed dialogue between purchasers and providers.

These payment innovations operate in different health systems and all come with their own specific challenges, but for policy makers, a number of important lessons should be considered:

Use payment systems to drive strategic objectives in health

- Align payment systems with health policy objectives. Payers need to be more innovative and providers should be rewarded for what they deliver – not simply what they can do.
- Encourage further experimentation. Add-on payments, bundled payments and population-based payment show promise, but more needs to be learnt about why some initiatives perform better than others.

Design payment innovations

- Draw on evidence-based guidelines to make tariff setting transparent, which will also encourage adherence to treatment protocols and more standardised care.
- Use clear, scientific-based criteria to identify patient populations for the payment innovation – for example high-risk patients or those with complex needs.
- Encourage quality targets to be based on best practice guidelines defined by institutions in charge of defining good practices for the payment innovation. Use a wide set of quality measures to make care delivery and performance more transparent for payers.
- Build-up IT system capability for data needs, such as measure individual costs items to define bundled tariffs; record payments for billing purposes that are adaptable to alternative modes of payment; integrate data that span across levels of care to inform price setting and identify high-cost patients in more complex payment innovations; record performance measures; and train staff to cope with new IT requirements.

Implement payment innovations

- Target stakeholders from the start and keep them engaged in the payment reform with a focus on building consensus about objectives, reporting and quality requirements, and mitigate concerns relating to exposure to financial risk among providers.
- Strike a balance between better data, data reporting and added administrative burden so as to reduce provider resistance to the change in payment.

Evaluate payment innovations

- Pilot experimentation to adjust incentives to providers and to mitigate possible unintended consequences before scaling up payment reform.
- Evaluate the payment innovation on a systematic basis through independent evaluations and build in systematic monitoring and feedback to providers to strengthen provider support to payment changes and accountability.

Assessment and recommendations

Predominant health care provider payment methods in OECD countries have been slow to reform and have often not rewarded value

Most often, health care providers are paid in the same way they always have been, using the traditional, dominant payment methods common across OECD health systems. Yet, these ways of paying providers – through fee-for-service (FFS), capitation, salary, global budget or more recently diagnosis-related groups (DRG) – are often poorly aligned with contemporary health system priorities. Rather than giving incentives to providers to improve quality, or deliver care more efficiently, "traditional" payment methods come with built-in incentives leading to undesirable behaviours, for instance over-provision of services or inattention to clinical need.

Traditional payment systems are particularly challenged by the shift in care needs that many OECD health systems are currently confronted with. Ageing societies and changes in life styles such as unhealthy diet and physical inactivity have led to a rise in the prevalence of chronic conditions. In addition, more and more patients now suffer from multiple morbidities. Traditionally, payment systems do little to support these new care models, as health service provision is predominantly financed in a "silo". Frequently, this results in fragmentation of care with poor patient experience and poor health outcomes.

This publication analyses some of the recent trends in provider payment reforms, the backgrounds for their implementations and the success of these payment innovations at leveraging intended policy goals. The innovations in payment mechanisms explored in this publication include add-on payments paid on top of existing payment methods, bundled payments, and population-based payments – drawing on latest evidence from OECD countries. They focus mainly on primary care and hospitals but in some cases can also stretch to rehabilitative care, long-term care and even pharmacies. The success of these payment innovations in achieving their policy goals – be that efficiency, quality, access, or otherwise – is considered, and potential lessons for health systems in other countries are drawn out.

Several countries have innovated provider payment mechanisms to address unwanted incentives of traditional mechanisms

Because health providers respond to financial incentives, all traditional modes of payment have specific strengths and weaknesses when it comes to meeting policy objectives. These also depend on the setting in which they are used, and other policy measures that can affect care delivery and utilisation.

For example, FFS payments typically incentivise providers to increase their clinical activity and as a result the associated costs. Capitation payments controls costs better but can encourage providers to deliver less health care than optimal for patients. Global budgets, too, control total costs, but may lead to access problems and waiting times. DRG payments focus on technical efficiency and reduce average length of stay but they also encourage hospitals to increase the number of patients.

The strengths and weaknesses of traditional payment systems in their "pure" form broadly let to three policy responses: i) blending payment methods to counterbalance their individual shortcomings; ii) adapting traditional modes of payment in an intelligent way; iii) developing new innovative ways to pay providers.

Blended payment systems and adaptations of traditional payment methods (Box 0.1) have worked well to attach specific health policy objectives to delivery, or to balance the negative and positive incentives of different payment mechanisms.

Box 0.1. Blending payment systems and adaptations of traditional payment methods

In primary care, the vast majority of OECD countries use blended forms of payments, for example combining capitation with FFS payments. Blended payments can mean that different payment mechanisms are applied to different primary care providers, or individual providers being paid through a blended mix of payment types.

Blended payments are less widely used for outpatient specialist care where the predominant payment method is FFS. Nevertheless some countries such as Sweden and the United Kingdom have incorporated blended forms of payment, such as global budgets along with combinations of pay-for-performance (P4P) and additional payments.

In inpatient care, blended payment systems are the norm. A mix of payment schemes can mean a combination of DRG and global budgets but can also include FFS payments for certain procedures, per-diem rates or line-item remuneration (less common). In public hospitals, DRGs and global budgets are most commonly used. A number of countries have moved towards case-based payment to meet specific health policy objectives to replace global budgets (Greece, Ireland), FFS (Korea) or per diems (Israel).

A second response is to adapt traditional payment systems. In primary care, nearly all OECD countries that use capitation adjust the payment for risk factors to discourage skimping of care and "cherry-picking" – that means the selection of positive risks – by providers. Risk factors include age, gender, health status, utilisation of services geographical or socioeconomic factors.

Global budgets have evolved beyond resource-based or historical budgets. In some countries budget allocation is also adjusted for risk factors (e.g. age, gender) to make it more equitable and transparent. Hospital budget allocation based on case-mix as measured via DRGs can help to benchmark hospitals and incentivise the efficient use of hospital resources. The introduction of volume thresholds can put a limit to spending increases. They are used in primary care for FFS or inpatient care for case-based payment by a number of OECD countries. Activity over a defined threshold is either rewarded at a reduced tariff or not remunerated at all.

Source: Authors' compilation.

Recently, some health systems have embarked on more innovative changes designed to improve care co-ordination, improve delivery for patient populations with complex health needs that span across levels of care, with an increased focus on quality metrics for monitoring and performance.

The analysed innovations can be broadly clustered into three distinct payment trends (Figure 0.1).

1. Add-on payments – ex post or ex ante – are made on top of existing payment methods for co-ordinating activities (as seen in France and Germany); or pay-for-performance (P4P) – focussed on improving quality of care implemented in many countries (e.g. Portugal and Norway) (Chapter 2).
2. Bundled payments; which can either refer to episode-based payments for specific activities of acute care based on best practice or following clinical pathways (e.g. England and Sweden) or payments for the care of chronic conditions that include

quality requirements across delivery settings (e.g. diabetes, HIV/AIDS), as seen in the Netherlands and Portugal (Chapter 3).

3. Population-based payment cover a wide range of services by various providers who are encouraged to control costs and meet quality standards (e.g. United States, Germany and Spain) (Chapter 4).

Figure 0.1. Innovative payment schemes in OECD countries

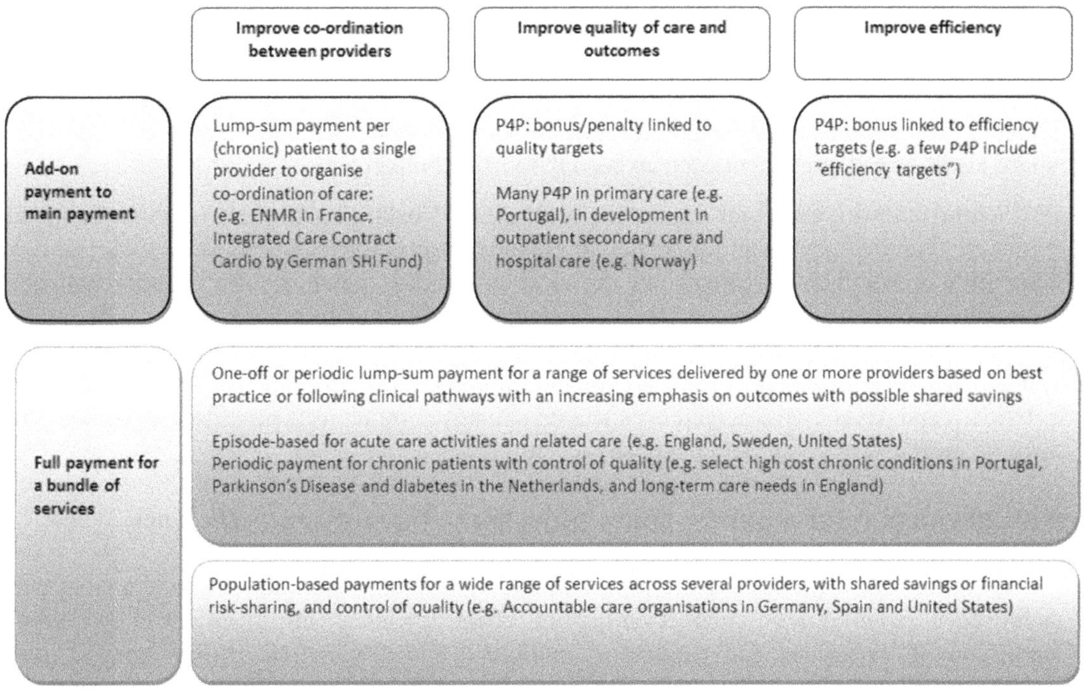

Source: Authors' compilation

Add-on payments are usually fairly easy to introduce as they are applied on top of existing payment methods. They can be made ex post or ex ante and are most frequently used to foster co-ordination of care, or to improve quality of care or efficiency and in many cases add-on payments pursue more than one of these goals. Add-on incentives predominantly aimed at improving co-ordination of care activities frequently take the form of FFS or lump-sum payments covering pre-defined activities for a period of time. Pay-for-performance (P4P) is typically an add-on payment to promote evidence-based and preventive services that are linked to specific "targets". P4P schemes are generally more sophisticated than add-on payments for co-ordination. P4P schemes have tended to focus on quality of care but can also have elements to improve efficiency (e.g. more efficient prescription of generics).

Bundled payments for acute care episodes are widely used in hospitals. Recent developments are of two kinds. First, some countries have extended episode-based payments to include pre- and post-surgery activities in the bundle. Second, and more recently, some countries have moved away from pricing case payments at the average cost of provision to introduce a more normative dimension that reflect evidence-based guidelines. The bundled payment of a number of different activities into one single payment for chronic conditions stretches beyond the inpatient sector is also relatively recent. A single tariff is calculated and is based on information from clinical guidelines to reflect activities covered in the care pathway.

Population-based payment targets groups of providers or management organisations responsible for the delivery of all – or the vast majority of – health care services for a defined group of the population. These entities are frequently referred to as Accountable Care Organizations (ACOs) following the adoption of this terminology in the United States. In this model, provider groups and payers agree on a "virtual budget" as a benchmark for a range of predefined services. The actual payment to providers is done through traditional payment mechanism such as capitation or FFS. Providers are encouraged to improve efficiency by the prospect to keep a share of savings generated for the payers if they can keep costs below an agreed benchmark value while meeting pre-defined quality criteria (referred to as a shared-savings contract). In some models, provider groups also have to share losses in case treatment costs exceed the virtual budget.

While innovative add-on payments such as P4P expose providers to little financial exposure, bundled payments for particular episodes expose providers to more financial risk than FFS or per diem payments. In the case of bundled payments for chronic patients, providers encounter the risk that chronic patients seek out health providers more often than envisaged when calculating the bundled tariff. Population-based bundled payments carry more risk where providers receive a capitated amount. The financial risk is softened when providers and payers have agreed on a shared savings contract as it permits the providers to take on more risk without being exposed to "full risk".

Innovative payment reform pursue policy objectives of quality and efficiency

A framework for assessing the policy impact of recent innovations considers what was achieved in terms of policy impact on quality, efficiency, costs, improvement in process of care and in outcomes for patients. Conditions under which a policy change was implemented are also considered. This includes stakeholder involvement, whether an adoption of the payment scheme is compulsory for payers and providers, whether the payment reform was a stand-alone reform or embedded in larger health policy reform, the administrative burden of the policy, how tariffs are set and whether data collection are used to inform price setting. Whether the reform was evaluated is a final key feature considered.

Key characteristics of selected payment innovations are presented in Table 0.1. Payment policies differ in the type and range of services they incentivise stretching from primary care to secondary care and beyond. The payment policies may target all patients or specific chronic populations or patients requiring certain acute care interventions. Providers involved include hospitals or a group of different health professionals.

A summary of the impact of different payment innovations are shown in Table 0.2 and Table 0.3. These show that many of the innovations have met policy objectives – improved quality and generated savings. The policy design of successful innovations predominantly involved transparent criteria for tariff setting and identifying the patient population. The implementation tended to focus on wide stakeholder engagement to catalyse buy-in. Evaluation of payment innovations were built into the policy, and many were experimented as pilots. The innovations had spill-over effects that led to increased data collection to expand the knowledge base on quality metrics and performance. However, there have been challenges including the complexity of the payment policy, increased administrative burden for providers and the reluctance among some providers to bear more financial risk.

Table 0.1. Key characteristics of payment reform in selected OECD countries

	Add-on payments				Episode-of-care or chronic condition payment							Population-based payment		
Country	DEU	FRA	PRT	NOR	USA	ENG	ENG	SWE	PRT	NLD	NLD	USA	DEU	ESP
Type and name of payment reform	Add-on co-ordination (Cardio-Integral)	Add-on co-ordination (ENMR)	Add-on payment (P4P) in primary care	Add-on payment (P4P) in hospitals	Bundled payment for acute care episodes cardiac and orthopedic care (ACE)	Best practice tariffs in hospitals (BPT)	Maternity care pathway	Bundled payment for an episode of care (SVEUS)	Bundled payment for select chronic conditions	Bundled payment for Parkinson's Disease	Bundled payment for diabetes, vascular risk management, COPD)	Medicare ACO	Gesundes Kinzigtal (GK)	Ribera Salud (Alzira)
Basket of services covered by innovation	Check-up, monitoring, patient preparation for invasive treatment, co-ordination	Co-ordinating activities by health professionals and health education	Primary care services, nursing services, home visits	All inpatient services	37 inpatient cardiac and orthopaedic procedures	50 clinical areas of hospital activities (e.g. stroke, hip fracture, cataract surgery)	Ante-natal, delivery and post-natal care	Spine surgery and follow-up care for two years	Outpatient treatment, diagnostic, therapeutic exams	Primary care, secondary care, tertiary care	Primary care and select specialist care	Primary care, secondary care plus other	Primary care, secondary care plus other	Primary care, secondary care plus other
Patient population (conditions/episode)	Cardio-vascular disease patients living in Saxony insured by AOK plus	Patients who attend one of the three multidisciplinary structures	Patients registed with the Family Health Unit	All inpatients	Patients requiring an inpatient stay for select cardiac or orthopaedic procedures	Patients requiring select hospital services (e.g. stroke, hip fracture, cataract surgery)	Pregnant women	Patients requring spine surgery	HIV/AIDS and other select high cost chronic rare conditions	Parkinson's disease	Type 2 diabetic patients, vascular risk management and COPD	All patients receiving most of their treatment by provider organised in ACO	All registered patients	All patients in health area
Providers involved	GPs and specialists, outpatient clinic of hospital	A mix of health professionals work together (e.g. doctors, midwives, nurses, pharmacists)	GPs, primary care nurses, and auxiliary staff	Four hospital regions comprised of public secondary care providers, and contracted private hospitals	Hospitals and physicians belonging to a facility in each participating site	Public hospitals	Public hospitals and midwifery teams, and birth centres	Public hospitals	Public hospitals	17 types of health professionals	Care groups of providers typically managed by GPs that include other health professionals (e.g. nurses)	GPs, specialist, hospitals, rehabilitation facilities, nursing homes	Provider network led by GPs	Hospital as lead provider but also health centres and outpatient clinics

Source: Authors' compilation.

Table 0.2. Assessment of payment reform in selected OECD countries

	Add-on payments				Bundled payments							Population-based payments		
Country	DEU	FRA	PRT	NOR	USA	ENG	ENG	SWE	PRT	NLD	NLD	USA	DEU	ESP
Type and name of payment reform	Add-on co-ordination (Cardio-Integral)	Add-on co-ordination (ENMR)	Add-on payment (P4P) in primary care	Add-on payment (P4P) in hospitals	Bundled payment for acute care episodes cardiac and orthopedic care (ACE)	Best practice tariffs in hospitals (BPT)	Maternity care pathway	Bundled payment for an episode of care (SVEUS)	Bundled payment for select chronic conditions	Bundled payment for Parkinson's Disease (ParkinsonNet)	Bundled payment for diabetes (select chronic conditions)	Medicare (ACO)	Gesundes Kinzigtal (GK)	Ribera Salud (Alzira)
Assessment of policy impact Achievement in terms of policy objective														
Quality	+	+	+	Evaluation due later	+	+/-	Evaluation not yet available	+	+	+ (before payment reform)	+	+/-	+/-	+
Savings	+	+	+	Evaluation due later	+		Reduction in caesarean section rate but savings evaluation not yet available	+	+	+ (before payment reform)	-	+/-	+	+
Unintended consequences										Competition concern		Best performing ACO can lose revenues		Contract renegotiation

Source: Authors' compilation.

Table 0.3. Conditions of payment reform in selected OECD countries

	Add-on payments				Bundled payments							Population-based payments		
Country	DEU	FRA	PRT	NOR	USA	ENG	ENG	SWE	PRT	NLD	NLD	USA	DEU	ESP
Type and name of payment reform	Add-on co-ordination (Cardio-Integral)	Add-on co-ordination (ENMR)	Add-on payment (P4P) in primary care	Add-on payment (P4P) in hospitals	Bundled payment for acute care episodes cardiac and orthopedic care (ACE)	Best practice tariffs in hospitals (BPT)	Maternity care pathway	Bundled payment for an episode of care (SVEUS)	Bundled payment for select chronic conditions	Bundled payment for Parkinson's Disease (ParkinsonNet)	Bundled payment for diabetes (select chronic conditions)	Medicare (ACO)	Gesundes Kinzigtal (GK)	Ribera Salud (Alzira)
Conditions for implementation														
Payment reform embedded in larger policy reform	+	+	+	-	+	+	+	+	+	-	+	+	+	+
Stakeholder participation in policy development			+	+	+	+	+	+	+	+	+			
Payer participation	Voluntary for SHI funds	Mandatory payments by SHI	Dependent on provider take up	Applied to all hospital regions	Mandatory	Mandatory	Mandatory	Mandatory	Mandatory	Voluntary	Voluntary	Mandatory for Medicare	Voluntary for SHI funds	Mandatory for public payer in some regions
Provider participation	Voluntary	Voluntary	Voluntary	Mandatory	Voluntary	Mandatory	Mandatory	Voluntary	Voluntary	Voluntary	Voluntary	Voluntary	Voluntary	Voluntary
Administrative Burden						+	+			+	+	+		+
Data collection and use			New data and existing	Existing data	New and existing data	Existing data	New and existing data	Existing data	EHR established	New and existing data	New and existing data	New and existing data	New and existing data	
How are tariffs set?	Negotiated by SHI funds and providers	Individual tariff depend on staff size of setting and number of patients, the total amount available for ENMR set at national level	Add-on payment based on nationally established indicators, and negotiated bonuses with local commissioner	Around 0.5% of the block grant budget allocated to the (4) regional hospital associations ithrough the P4P scheme	Bundle of Medicare Part A and Medicare Part B services and negotiated at each site	Tariff reflects best practice extends current system of average costs	Total costs of antenatal, delivery and postnatal care	Tariffs set to reflect clinical guidelines and can include follow-up, warranty payment and outcome information	According to clinical guidelines such as follow up, number of medical appointments, diagnostic exams, and therapeutic regimen	Capitated payment currently being piloted	Negotiated between care groups and insurers while sub-contractors negotiate their own payments	Benchmark based on past spending and adjusted annually for total Medicare spending trend	Benchmark based on SHI funds reimbursement from risk-structure equalisation	Negotatied capitated amount, adjusted annually with total regional health budget increase
Independent evaluation of reform	+	+	+		+	+		+	+	+	+	+	+	-

Source: Authors' compilation.

Add-on payments for co-ordination can work across different levels of care, but are not always linked to cost savings

Add-on payments – both ex ante and ex post – are being used to incentivise co-ordination of health services across different levels of care, as seen in France with the introduction of the "*Expérimentations de nouveaux modes de rémunération*" (ENMR), an ex ante payment to multidisciplinary structures, and in Germany for patients with cardiovascular disease (the "Cardio-Integral" programme) via a payment ex post to individual providers. In both countries, add-on payments represent additional sources of revenue for providers, but account for a relatively small share of total provider income, 5% or less.

Assessment of policy impact: Improvements in quality and lower costs for co-ordinating care

In both France and Germany, add-on payments are associated with an improvement in the quality of care provided and reductions in health spending, although it is difficult to establish clear causality. In France, the multi-disciplinary structures achieve better results for nearly all care indicators (e.g. diabetes care processes; prevention and efficient prescription) with the most significant improvements in controlling HbA1c levels than traditional practices – although they were already performing better before the introduction of the ENMR. Costs in multidisciplinary structures were between 0.5% and 2.3% lower than in traditional practices. However, the cost differences pre-date the introduction of the payment scheme in France.

Similarly, positive results were found with the Cardio-Integral programme in Germany for patients with cardiovascular disease. There has been a reduction in repeat examination and better patient-centred collaboration between doctors. About 89% of patients acknowledge better co-operation between GP and cardiologist and 65% of patients report an improvement in their health status after enrollment. After higher initial set-up costs, the programme was able to generate savings after nearly five years. The estimated annual savings were about EUR 96 per enrolled patient due to improved drug therapy and better post-acute treatment, which helped to bring down inpatient costs for invasive interventions and heart failure. However, it is difficult to separate out the contribution of the add-on payment provided under the "Cardio-Integral" contract as it overlaps with a Disease Management Program (DMP) for cardio-vascular diseases.

Conditions for implementation: Add-on payments for co-ordination are part of broader health reforms, easy to implement but limited in scope

In both countries, the introduction of add-on payments were part of *broader health reforms* which helped implementation. In France, the implementation of the ENMR complemented other health policy reforms. For example, the introduction of the P4P scheme CAPI/ROSP[1] was introduced around the same time. In Germany, the Cardio-Integral contract is an application of a change in the federal social code allowing selective contracting between individual health insurance funds and individual or groups of health providers for care delivery models across sectors.

Overall, add-on payments for co-ordination are relatively easy to implement and do not seem to face significant provider resistance. They generally require few IT investments and data exchanges. The administrative burden of these innovations can be expected to be comparably small. Yet the scope of these incentives is limited, as they focus on the improvement of co-operation of health professionals within and across provider settings and incentivise specific behaviours at specific points of the care pathway.

Add-on payments to reward quality have led to quality improvements however it is difficult to separate their impact from those of the other initiatives

Add-on payments which reward quality and performance, known as P4P also sit alongside existing payments systems. The main difference between P4P and the add-on payment for co-ordination is that P4P payments are focussed on the degree of achievement of specific defined objectives by providers or practitioners. As such, they are systematically applied ex post. P4P schemes typically promote evidence-based and preventive services that are linked to specific "targets" and have emerged as one potential lever to address some of the shortcomings of traditional payments of FFS, capitation, and salary.

P4P schemes are now widespread across OECD countries, and beyond. In 2012, nearly two-thirds of OECD countries reported having at least one P4P scheme in place. The largest number of P4P programmes is found in primary care but P4P are also spreading to specialists and acute hospitals. In primary care, bonuses are paid most frequently for the achievement of targets relating to preventive care and the management of chronic diseases, less often for the uptake of IT initiatives, patient satisfaction or efficient care provision (e.g. share of generic medicines prescribed). In the majority of countries, bonus payments are made to the individuals based on the achievement of absolute targets. In hospitals, P4P targets relate most commonly to patient experience, clinical outcomes and the use of appropriate processes. In most OECD countries, hospital performance is measured either as absolute targets or observed changes over time.

In Ontario, Canada, P4P was introduced to primary care practitioners as part of a wider diversification of payment mechanisms. In Portugal, P4P was introduced as a payment component for medical staff that work in newly established models of primary care – Family Health Units (FHU). Norway has introduced a P4P component to payment in Norway's four hospital regions to encourage greater policy attention towards patient-centred care and increased emphasis on systematic quality improvement, patient safety and reduction in adverse events.

Beyond these examples, performance-based payment is used for specific patient groups as in the case of diabetes in Australia, France or Germany, and also being introduced in more diverse care settings, for example long-term care in the United States, or again public health and prevention outside of GP practices such as for delivery of vaccination services or smoking cessation in pharmacies in the United Kingdom.

Assessment of policy impact: Some quality improvement but no clear breakthrough in performance

Systematic reviews tentatively suggest a positive impact of P4P programmes on performance, but evidence on the impact of P4P on health outcomes remains limited and inconclusive. No clear "breakthrough" in performance improvement can be clearly linked to the introduction of a P4P scheme, although improvements on some indicators, mainly relating to quality are found for a number of P4P schemes.

This is true, for example, in Australia, Canada, France, Germany, Norway and Portugal, where there is some possible positive influence of P4P schemes on provider performance. In Portugal, the reform in primary care, in which a P4P component was introduced, has shown improvements in care quality, patient and practitioner satisfaction in the newly created FHU models compared to the traditional solo practices. In Ontario, Canada, the voluntary P4P programme appears to be a popular alternative for GP practices to using exclusively FFS and is tied to certain practice and staffing requirements, for instance patient registration goals and minimum staffing and staff profile standards. In Germany there is some modest impact of the diabetes Disease Management Programmes on quality, while trend effects make it difficult to isolate the effect of *Rémunération sur Objectifs de Santé Publique* in France or the Practice Incentive Program in Australia. In some settings, P4P schemes have sought to redistribute or redirect existing resources (e.g. in Canada, Norway and Portugal) while in others, there were significant injections of new funds (QOF in the United Kingdom and Turkey's "Family medicine performance based contracting" scheme). However, there is no conclusive evidence of any P4P programme which has been cost saving.

In addition, P4P programmes have brought about some other important system benefits. A review of twelve P4P programmes concluded that while the impact of P4P has been relatively minimal, the P4P programmes improved the clarification of the goals of providers, improved purchasing processes, better measurement of provider activity and performance, and more informed dialogue between purchasers and providers.

The successes of P4P payment reform need to be seen in context of other dimensions, such organisational change (e.g. Portugal, Canada) or a broader reform agenda on quality improvement (Norway). In instances where P4P programmes are implemented alongside non-financial incentives such as performance feedback or public reporting, some of the potential performance improvement may be attributable to the alternative incentives. It is difficult to separate out the influence of the change in payment method from other factors, such as the influence of self-selection – that is providers who sign up for a voluntary schemes may already be performing better, and simply get paid for what they are doing anyway (in Canada, and Portugal), underlying trends in improving quality of care (in Australia or France), or indeed changes or improvement to the way that relevant data is recorded and reported. Moreover, P4P payments may encourage overprovision of unnecessary services covered by the scheme and thus need to be designed so they do not discourage non-incentivised activities. Given that the P4P component is usually small, the dominant payment system has the potential to either undo the effects of P4P programmes, or reinforce them where the goal of both incentive structures aligns. Despite all reported examples of P4P for health providers sitting alongside other payment mechanisms, research on the interaction between P4P and the dominant payment system is quite weak.

There have not, to date, been comprehensive independent reforms of either the P4P programme in Canada and Norway. An evaluation is expected from Norway in the near future. A better understanding of the successes and failures of P4P as an approach, and individual P4P programmes, would be greatly advanced by more thorough independent evaluations of existing programmes.

Conditions for implementation: P4P prioritise quality improvements, motivate providers around data collection however they are complicated to administer

P4P payments sometimes have been embedded in broader reforms. In Norway, the P4P programme in the hospital sector came as part of a broader reform on systematic quality improvement. In other cases, P4P programmes were linked to organisational or financial changes (meeting certain pre-requisites around quality of information or indicators). In Portugal, P4P was part of a broader organisational change to primary care, and a shift from facility-level payment based on salaries to mixed payment including salary, capitation and P4P. Likewise in Canada, P4P schemes introduced for primary care physicians were tied closely to organisational changes, notably requirements that physicians work in group models and that after-hours care be provided.

The introduction of P4P schemes can motivate providers towards *better and broader data collection*. While in Norway and Portugal pre-existing rich data infrastructures have supported the introduction of P4P, it remains the case that in many countries good building blocks for P4P – notably appropriate performance measures – are missing. Data improvements have come through direct incentives for providers to invest in information infrastructure (IT, electronic medical records) as in Australia PIP, California IHA, and France ROSP/CAPI, or related to minimum IT standards being a criterion for participation in the P4P scheme, for instance in the UK QOF. The data sources used in P4P programmes will also have an impact on administrative burden; if pre-existing data sources are used, as in Norway and Portugal, the introduction of incentives tied to the data is unlikely to entail new data reporting burdens, but may help improve reporting rate and fidelity.

However, P4P schemes are more *complex to administer* as they require data systems for collection, measurement and the calculation of rewards. Most P4P have been using process indicators or intermediate outcome indicators, with a more limited number of P4P programmes including patient experience measures or negative penalties. The P4P schemes in Portugal and Canada are in large part focussed on clinical processes, and incentivising care that is consistent with best practice guidelines, but also cover access and efficiency domains. Indicators of quality also include outcome indicators, such as intermediate outcomes – controlled blood pressure, blood sugar, cholesterol – are used for instance in the California IHA programme or the QOF in the United Kingdom, and in the Portuguese FHUs. Norway's hospital-based P4P programme includes non-intermediate outcome measures, notably cancer mortality. Patient experience is an important outcome indicator of quality and a potential lever for quality improvement (e.g. Portugal and Norway, as well as England, Israel and Korea).

To measure performance, absolute, relative and competitive targets can be quite complex and are used across different P4P schemes, and also within single schemes. In Portugal, indicators are used to meet absolute target thresholds, while in Norway absolute and relative rankings are used. A number of payment schemes use absolute measures (e.g. proportion of hypertensive patients) to set a minimum standard, which is then supplemented with or sits alongside differently adjusted targets. Negative penalties are used in Norway's P4P programme where payment is capped, and covers a small part of the block grant each region receives annually. Since 2008, the Centres for Medicare and Medicaid Services (CMS) use similar negative incentives for hospital performance in the United States where payments can be withheld for certain avoidable conditions, including "never" events and other complications that were not present on admission such as hospital-acquired infections, or have been shown to be largely preventable.

Bundled payments are used widely and show improved quality, however they require sophisticated IT systems

Bundled payments for health care are being used in several OECD countries. The new forms of bundled payments discussed in this publication refer to innovations in bundled activities grouped into a single tariff that go beyond simple DRG payments. They can cover both acute care and chronic conditions.

There are a number of examples of bundled payments for acute care episodes from the United States and include Medicare's initiative for inpatient cardiac and orthopaedic procedures launched in 2009 (ACE) as well as private sector initiatives such as ProvenCare for coronary artery bypass surgery. Other initiatives include the PROMETHEUS model covering episodes-of-care and chronic conditions and the Integrated Healthcare Association (IHA) for orthopaedic surgery, both of which encountered problems with implementation.

The United Kingdom (England) developed best practice tariffs (BPTs) implemented in 2010 for four clinical areas (e.g. hip fracture, stroke) and now cover 50 areas and more recently a bundled payment for maternity care was introduced. Sweden launched a nationwide collaboration to develop bundled payments focussing on 8 areas covering both episodes of care (e.g. hip replacement, spine surgery) and chronic conditions (e.g. diabetes).

For chronic conditions, Portugal launched a series of pilot bundle payments in 2007 for select high cost chronic conditions (e.g. HIV/AIDS, multiple sclerosis) that require a medical consultation and certain outpatient services where the tariffs are set to follow clinical guidelines. The Netherlands established a bundle payment for patients with select chronic conditions (type 2 diabetes, COPD and vascular risk management) where "care groups" are contracting partners for insurers for the provision of pre-defined activities within a year. For patients with Parkinson's disease, regional networks of different health providers (ParkinsonNet) began in 2004 to first improve the delivery of care (primary, secondary and tertiary settings) for their patients while maintaining the traditional modes of payment for service delivery. The second phase of collaboration, currently not yet fully implemented, involves developing a bundled payment including outcome information.

Assessment of policy impact: Bundled payments show quality improvements, generate savings, better patient satisfaction, but the gains depend on the condition or episode targeted for reform

Bundled payments based on best practice or adjusted according to quality indicators show some promise to achieve quality gains for episodes-of-care and chronic conditions. For acute conditions, a number of initiatives have seen reductions in readmission rates, complications and improved mortality figures for hip and knee replacement and bypass surgery as seen in the United States, England and Sweden. For other procedures, such as stroke, experimentations have not shown any quality improvements in England. In the case of chronic conditions, better performance and higher patient satisfaction have been detected in the Netherlands for diabetes and Parkinson's disease and better adherence to medication and treatment protocol were associated with the bundled payment for HIV in Portugal.

Costs were reduced in a number of instances for bypass surgeries and hip and knee replacements, mainly achieved by reductions in average length of stay and reduced number of readmissions as seen in the United States and Sweden. For example, the acute care demonstration (ACE) saved USD 319 per episode for a savings of USD 4 million in the United States. For bundled payments for chronic conditions average treatment costs for HIV were reduced in Portugal through better adherence to treatment plans but costs increased in the case of diabetes patients after the introduction bundled payments in the Netherlands (e.g. with a cost per patient of EUR 288) which may be partly be driven by delaying required specialist care – not included in the bundled tariffs.

Most of the bundled payment initiatives have undergone evaluations whether they are included explicitly as part of the policy process or not. There are no published evaluations for the maternity pathway bundled payment in England (United Kingdom). Currently, there are also no evaluations yet available for the bundled payment for Parkinson's disease as it has not been fully implemented.

Conditions for implementation: Stakeholder support led to improved protocols of care, along with a focus on outcome measurement and data collection, however, tariff setting can be complex, and increase the administrative burden

Stakeholder participation can catalyse the implementation of bundled payments as seen in England, Portugal, Sweden and the Netherlands, but continued support can be challenging as it may require balancing opposing interests between purchaser and provider. For example, there were successful negotiations between payer and provider to agree on discounted payment rates in the United States Medicare ACE demonstration. In other examples, clinicians were engaged in informing the tariffs as seen in England and Portugal. A wide group of stakeholders were involved at the outset in Sweden including local authorities, national specialist associations, national quality registries, patient associations as well as academia. In the Netherlands, while the bundled payment for diabetes was policy led, a bottom-up approach was taken for Parkinson's disease and driven by providers supported by patients and some health insurers. In this context, the move towards a bundled payment is the end result of restructuring of care processes and not the first step.

Stakeholder support also played a part in the organisational changes in the care delivery process. Health care providers intensified their collaboration – within and across settings – and a greater standardisation of care was achieved. Generally, this was facilitated and accompanied by the development of guidelines, the monitoring of cost and quality including feedback loops to providers. In Sweden, for example, the professional associations played a key role to develop new manuals and checklists along with the other stakeholders (e.g. local authorities) to standardise practise and establish benchmarks. Guidelines were reviewed and standardised protocols were established along with feedback monitoring systems as seen in the United States ACE demonstration and ProvenCare. Contracts between care groups and insurers were based on standardised protocols of care drawn from national guidelines for diabetes care in the Netherlands. Care standardisation is also an important element of the Parkinson networks in the Netherlands, even if they predate the introduction of the bundled payment. There, members of the network are required to meet a number of minimal standards (e.g. treating a minimum number of patients per year or the regular attendance of multi-disciplinary team meeting to discuss cases and stimulate collaboration).

Bundled payment also resulted in a shift of tasks across providers and even changes in the scope of practice and responsibilities of selected heath care professions as seen in the Netherlands. In the bundled payment for diabetes, practice nurses have taken on a more central role and carried most if not all the regular check-ups in GP practices, though it was reported this shift had already begun before the payment reform. Eye examinations were conducted outside the settings of ophthalmologists such as by optometrists or general practice laboratories.

The move towards bundled payments has been frequently tested *at a pilot stage* before being rolled out on a greater scale. This helped to verify whether changes in the payments system had the desired effects and allowed for adjusting incentives before general implementation. Portugal began a five-year pilot payment for HIV/AIDS in selected hospitals before expanding it nationwide two years later. The bundled payment for hip and knee surgery in Sweden laid the groundwork for a national collaboration to reform payment systems there. In the Netherlands, evaluations of the diabetes pilot were built into the policy process when the pilot was expanded nationwide in 2009. As an intermediate step, for paying for Parkinson's disease, a "lighter-version" which used budget allocation based on capitation for hospital care was piloted in 2014.

Furthermore, there is a growing *consideration of data on health outcomes* in bundled payment initiatives. Sweden is the most advanced in this regard where for spine surgery, 10% of the payment is related to patient's functionality post-surgery. In the Netherlands, the bundled payment for diabetes includes process and outcome indicators because the earlier contracts had limited provisions for justifying the content and quality of care. For Parkinson's disease, a set out of outcome indicators is collected to inform the bundle payment model which is currently under development.

Bundled payment has also led to further improvements in data systems and measurement. This includes integrated information systems in the Netherlands (diabetes bundled payment), and new data systems and data collections as seen in Portugal and in the Netherlands for Parkinson's disease. In others, there were monitoring systems to allow for rapid feedback as well as identifying anomalies as seen in Sweden. Even where payment reform was abandoned or not implemented, IT systems led to improvements in reporting (Denmark) and helped to identify data needs for measurement of quality and cost (PROMETHEUS in the United States).

However, *tariff setting for bundled payments can be complex*. It can include identifying and pricing of all services that constitute best practice along an evidence-based pathway, incorporating quality measures, and may refer to one single payment or are made up of several payments. In England, the pricing for some models under the Best Practice Tariff, includes a "base price" (which is lower than or equal to a tariff set for the conventional way of providing care, i.e. based on the national average of reported costs) and a "BPT component." Best practice tariffs can be higher or lower than national average costs, and are paid if best practice guidelines for treatment are followed. The BPT for fragility hip fracture, for example, is made up of a base tariff and a conditional payment, payable if a number of characteristics are achieved (e.g. time to surgery within 36 hours from arrival in an emergency department). In Sweden, the bundled payment for spine surgery includes the intervention, costs for pre and post-operative visits, rehabilitation as well as a warranty payment for complications. Here, historical costs were used to inform tariff setting. In the Netherlands, a single annual payment per patient is defined for standard diabetic care and bundled payment contracts are negotiated between health insurers and care groups.

Setting and managing these tariffs brings about new *additional administrative work*, both for payers and providers. To set tariffs, costs for separate activities within the bundled payment need to be identified. In case the payment incorporates quality metrics, process or outcome indicators need to be measured and reported. There may be issues around exchange of information between providers if a bundled payment reflects evidence-based treatment across providers. Finally, modifications to existing billing practice may require additional guidelines if more than one provider is involved.

In England, despite provider support towards BPT payments, the changes were challenging to implement and difficult to understand for providers. The Audit Commission recommended making price setting simpler and clearer with a more transparent explanation of the BPT payment models that should be reported alongside public reporting of quality of care. For diabetes care in the Netherlands, the quality of the data reporting among care groups was mixed and required standardisation as health insurance companies were also not always satisfied about the quality of the accountability information they received from care groups. Furthermore, there was poor IT integration between GPs and care groups requiring data to be entered twice into both IT systems. For the maternity bundled payment in England, there was an administrative burden relating to invoicing providers for their services as the complexity of information did not allow for the flow of confidential data, which made it difficult for finance departments to determine the lead provider for invoicing purposes.

Finally, *diverging interests and fear of financial risk can* impede implementation. Some bundled payment initiatives encountered different problems and were subsequently not implemented as envisaged. Agreement on bundle definitions was difficult to reach between providers and payers for the IHA bundle and in the PROMETHEUS project in the United States. In the latter case, the risk of financial exposure by providers contributed to low participation preventing an evaluation to take place. In the IHA demonstration, interests of participants diverged as health plans wanted to negotiate lower prices while hospitals wanted a higher level payment than under FFS. Other initiatives were abandoned after low provider participation as seen in the case of the bundled payment for diabetic care in Denmark. There, the financial incentive was too low to encourage GP participation. Even though additional funds were provided to implement an IT system, they were not seen to be sufficient.

Population-based payments have shown improvements in chronic disease management and preventive care and some savings, however they require a robust technical design

Population-based payments include provisions to make sure provider groups meet quality targets before they can benefit from any savings they generate. This distinguishes them from previous approaches, such as the managed-care contracts in the United States in the 1980s and 1990s or GP fundholding in the United Kingdom. These initiatives, too, shifted some of the financial risk onto providers, but they did not have any incentives to improve or maintain a minimum level of quality. Generally, the provider groups contracted to population-based payments are referred to as Accountable Care Organisations (ACOs) following the terminology of the largest experiment in the United States. In 2014, around 600 ACOs contracted by Medicare or private insurers provide care for about 20 million patients in the United States. First implemented in 2012, there are currently three types of Medicare ACO programmes operating: Medicare Shared Savings Programme (MSSP) ACO – mainly shared savings only; advanced Payment ACO (targets rural areas); and Pioneer ACO (most risk-involving for providers) – shared savings and losses. Smaller initiatives exist in Germany, for example in a rural area in South-Western Germany with a physician-led ACO (Gesundes Kinzigtal GmbH – GK) and in the Spanish region of Valencia where a private contractor (Ribera Salud Group) is accountable for primary and secondary care in several health areas including "Alzira". Providers are remunerated for the provision of services in the traditional way in all population-based payment models, which is mainly fee-for-service (United States, Germany). The Spanish contractors receive capitation payments to provide primary and secondary care.

Assessment of policy impact: Performance improved but not all generated savings

In the United States, both Pioneer ACOs and MSSP ACOs reported better performance than for benchmark Medicare beneficiaries. Pioneer ACOs improved their performance in 28 of the 33 quality measures in their second year of evaluation, particularly for the at-risk population which suggests that some progress in the co-ordination of care for patients with chronic conditions was made. For MSSP ACOs, patient experience improved including timely access to doctors, and patients were better informed by their primary care physician about specialty care. More time-robust findings exist for some longer-standing private ACOs. Over four years, improvements in quality were faster for those patients enrolled in ACOs contracted by Blue Cross Blue Shields (BCBS) for the Alternative

Quality Contract (AQC) in Massachusetts than for a control group. This refers to a better performance in process measures for ambulatory care in the area of chronic disease management, adult preventive care and paediatric care as well as intermediate outcome measures, such as blood pressure control. For a private ACO in Sacramento, hospital readmissions within 30 days decreased by 15% in the first year. Over the same period though, emergency department utilisation increased.

No quality targets are set as part of the GK contract in Germany, but evaluations found reduced mortality rates for those persons participating in the ACO model, and higher survival rates for chronic heart disease patients while a programme for the elderly showed improved in nutrition behaviour but no improvement in physical activity and no changes in health-related quality of life. Internal evaluations of hospitals attached to Ribera Salud in Spain showed significantly better results than for hospitals in the same region such as waiting times for emergency visits and external consultations are half that of the regional average.

On an aggregate level, ACOs slowed health spending growth for Medicare in the United States, but not all ACOs were able to generate savings, and among those that did, not all realised the minimum savings required to be eligible to keep part of the savings. Evaluations from the AQC in the private sector showed that saving on claims compared to the control groups could be realised in each of the four years but net savings (after programme costs) could only be realised in the fourth year. In Germany, GK kept their actual costs 6.6% below the benchmark budget in 2012 and these savings were shared between the two contracting health insurance funds and the ACO. In Spain, internal evaluations of Ribera Salud publish very large savings for the ACO in the health area of Alzira, with costs 25% lower than the average cost per inhabitant in Valencia but no external validation are available to confirm these figures.

Independent evaluations are embedded into the policy process as seen in Germany and the United States and are conducive to the overall acceptance by providers and patients as well as providing policy-makers with unbiased information. For example, the Medicare ACO programmes are regularly evaluated by independent researchers and results publically available. In Germany, evaluations are co-ordinated by an institute attached to the medical department of a university. Only in Spain, however, the impact of the ACO model on costs and quality of care has not been evaluated by an independent authority.

Conditions for implementation: Population-based payments were accompanied by voluntary participation and incentives to keep costs down and collect more comprehensive data, however they bring an added administrative burden

ACO implementation *depends on a robust technical design*. The size of the population assigned to an ACO varies widely between countries reflecting differences in multi-payer and single-payer health systems as well as the size of the pool of providers involved and differences in care organisation and delivery process. It is not possible to generalise whether there is an optimal population size of an ACO to be successful, but evidence from the United States suggests a minimum size of 25 000 to 50 000 enrollees would be needed to refinance needed investments, while results of the MSSP ACO after the first year showed that small, predominantly physician-led ACOs with less than 8 000 patients generated savings for Medicare which may indicate that smaller ACOs can implement changes in care delivery more quickly. The patient populations range from 5 000 and 50 000 in the United States, Germany has 9 400 covered in the GK contract while in Spain, 245 000 inhabitants of the health area Alzira are automatically assigned to the ACO. Furthermore, the provider composition of an ACO will strongly influence the care strategy the ACO will implement to reduce spending and improve care quality. Networks can be led by primary care providers (Germany), hospitals (Spain), or joint models. In the United States most ACOs are made up of medium-size hospital-physician groups or large systems with a high degree of integration delivering a wide range of services frequently including one or more post-acute facilities.

Implementation of population-based payments has gained traction in all countries because the payment reform was frequently part of a *wider health policy reform* including legislative/legal changes. In the United States, the creation of Medicare ACOs was included in the Patient Protection and Affordable Care Act (ACA) of 2010. ACOs are considered as one important tool to move away from a strict FFS scheme towards a payment system that rewards quality and value for Medicare beneficiaries. In Germany, integrated care contracts between individual insurers and individual providers were made legally possible in the early 2000s which allowed for the joint venture GK to contract two health insurers for the ACO model. In Spain, the implementation of the ACO model followed a change in national law to allow for private-public partnership in the health sector becoming effective in late 1990s.

Roll-out of the new model of payment and care provision started gradually in the United States. But many of their features were already tested before in earlier programmes (e.g. Physician Group Practice Demonstrations). For Germany, the GK can be considered as a pilot and the management company co-owning GK is currently planning to establish similar arrangements in other regions. The Alzira model in Spain has meanwhile been scaled up and by 2011 the Ribera Salud Group had implemented six population-based contracts in different areas of the region of Valencia.

Providers can freely decide *to participate* and apply for inclusion in the Medicare programme in the United States, or contracts are negotiated between payers and providers as seen in the private sector in the United States, in Germany (between insurers and a joint venture comprised of health providers and a management company) or Spain (between private contractors and regional health ministries). Patients have some choice as well. In both Medicare and the private sector in the United States, patients are "assigned" to an ACO if their doctor participates. Patients must be registered in Germany whereas in Spain, they are assigned to primary care providers but can choose specialist care in hospitals not managed by Ribera Salud.

All population-based payments include a focus on developing *strategies to keep cost down*, but they also give provider groups the autonomy to develop their own strategy. As a consequence, care models were rethought and pathways redesigned to make them more patient-centred with less fragmentation between the providers. The strategies focussed on improving care delivery in a number of ways such as care co-ordination for patients with chronic conditions, reducing hospitals readmission and emergency department visits (e.g. United States), preventive activities targeting patients with specific conditions and rational pharmacotherapy (e.g. Germany), attachment of a consultant physician to each health centre as a link to GPs facilitating the implementation of clinical guidelines and effectively reducing the number of inappropriate hospital referrals (Spain).

Sophisticated IT infrastructure is also vital for ACOs. In particular, bringing health care costs down requires good case management and the stratification of patients to identify those who benefit most from early interventions. These tasks are facilitated by electronic patient records and inter-operability of IT systems of different providers within an ACO, as well as by electronic management of appointment and referrals. Most successful arrangements use integrated IT systems that allow real-time monitoring of metrics which are connected to registries and public reporting systems. IT support is also required for the collection and submission of data to calculate quality indicators which are required in different ACO programmes. The hospitals associated with Ribera Salud in Valencia were reported to be the first public hospitals with a fully integrated electronic medical history system including medical notes, test results and imaging (NHS European Office, 2011). In some ACO models there is financial support for health providers to set up the required IT infrastructure, either from payers (e.g. Medicare in the Advance ACO model) or the ACO (GK in Germany).

However, the management of shared savings contracts can come with *considerable administrative burden* for participating providers as a result of contract managing and the measuring and reporting of cost and quality indicators. These issues seem to be most pronounced in the United States where ACOs that are contracted by Medicare in the Pioneer ACO programme, are actually encouraged to engage in similar contracts with other payers such as Medicaid or private insurers. For each payer, important elements of the ACO contracts can differ (e.g. risk-sharing models, quality indicators). One health provider network working with four different ACO arrangements was required to report on 219 different performance measures. In Spain, the establishment of a public private partnership contract in the health sector and its eventual re-negotiation appears to have been a rather complex endeavour. But unlike in the United States, Ribera Salud contracts only with a single payer.

Finally, there are *financial consequences* for ACOs and payers. Whether providers can get any additional financial reward depends on their ability to keep the costs below a benchmark budget. The benchmark budgets are defined by the size and characteristics of the population and by a range of services which vary between the different ACO models. Past spending is an important element in defining benchmark values as seen in the United States (e.g. Medicare ACOs are adjusted for spending growth). In Germany, the benchmark is defined annually by the Central Health Fund via the Risk-Structure-Compensation mechanism[2] to keep the cost below a "virtual budget". In Spain, a capitated amount was negotiated between ACO and the regional health ministry and is adjusted annually taking into account the total regional health budget increase. The financial exposure to payers will depend on a variety of factors such as whether there is a cap or maximum pay-out, and the rules for distributing the savings between the payer and the ACO. ACOs share savings without exposure to losses in a one-sided contract (seen in Germany and a common model in the United States); or exposure to losses in two-sided contracts (United States and Spain). ACOs typically use earned savings to invest in infrastructure or share them between individual providers.

Unintended financial consequences were observed in Spain because the initial contract (only covering secondary care) was not financial viable and had to be renegotiated. The regional ministry had to change it to include primary care resulting in an increase in the capitation rate. In the United States, the limitation of ACOs to population-based payments only for the Medicare population can have negative financial consequences for providers. The improved care processes implemented as part of ACO model can benefit patients covered under other schemes whose payment contracts did not foresee a possibility to earn savings. Other unintended consequences include low staff satisfaction with working conditions and skimping of care for some chronic patient groups as reported in Spain, and shifting of care where one successful ACO (Sacramento) in the United States successfully reduced hospital admissions and readmission in their first year but at the expense of increased use of emergency departments.

Conclusions

Currently, the most common ways health care providers are paid do not do enough to encourage high-quality care in OECD health systems. These traditional methods of paying providers are at odds with current health system priorities of changing epidemiology, care models for an ageing population, patients with complex health needs and scarce resources.

Many OECD countries have tried to adapt existing methods of payment to address some of their shortcomings. Some countries have embarked on more significant changes to their payment systems. This report has looked at three main types of such payment innovations: add-on payments, bundled payments and population-based payment. These innovations are underway in all types of health systems – for instance, where health care coverage is residence-based as well as those with insurance coverage. They also happen in health systems that are closely organised at a central level as well as in the countries where health systems are organised on a regional level. Their scope, though, differ. For example, add-on payments (either for co-ordination or as P4P) are more limited in scope, targeting particular activities or performance measures. P4Ps are provider-specific but can target various performance domains for each provider. Bundled payments for acute care episodes are more hospital-specific. The bundled payment for chronic conditions, conversely, can span across more settings. Finally, population-based bundling stretches across providers as they are collectively responsible for the provision of a wide range of pre-defined services.

The three types of payment innovations aim to better align provider incentives with health policy objectives and illustrate a significant departure from past ways to pay for health care. While evidence is limited, the evidence so far is that these innovations show promise. Importantly, these changes in payment systems reflect a growing use of evidence-based approaches that help move health systems towards greater accountability for patient's outcomes. The key findings from this report are as follows:

Innovations in payments are leading to efficiency gains as seen in reduction in costs or a slow-down in health spending growth, helping providers deliver greater quality care and benefitting many patients

- Add-on payments, bundled payments and population-based payment have shown to deliver better value and patients are benefitting thanks to these changes. Such innovative payment systems are increasingly using data on health care quality and health outcomes to inform tariff setting and report performance.
- Add-on payments contributed to better co-ordination of care, and improved quality of care such as chronic disease management, while controlling costs.
- The effects of P4P schemes are generally positive on quality-related processes but do not necessarily improve health outcomes. However, they can generate system-wide benefits such as introducing better data collection or leading to more informed dialogues between purchasers and providers.
- Bundled payments have led to improved quality of care, such as a reduction in readmissions, improved patient adherence and better patient satisfaction, while also generating savings in some areas.
- Population-based payments have shown potential to overcome fragmentation of care in the majority of cases leading to improved chronic disease management, preventive care and even outcomes, while reducing spending in a good number of cases.

Payment innovation have encouraged greater accountability for outcomes

- Providers involved in payment innovations are willing to accept rewarding models that entail more financial risk for them. This shift has been particularly successful where providers have more flexibility in care organisation.
- Payers have been more actively engaged in shaping modes of payment in countries where they are allowed to play a more strategic purchasing role. Policy levers emphasised evidence, systematic evaluation, provider engagement, and robust IT systems.
- As payment policies draw on evidence-based practice to inform price setting, payment innovation reforms have contributed to standardisation of processes, increased provider collaboration, and improved data collection. Ultimately, these changes encourage evidence-based approaches grounded on higher accountability for outcomes.

Payment innovations are not without challenges to manage carefully

- Innovations can add to the administrative burden.
- Bundled and population-based payments demand more full-scale reform and are more complex in design.
- Providers adapt their behaviour to incentives embodied in payment systems and they may eventually also learn to "game" them.
- Where additional reforms were introduced, it has been more difficult to attribute any observed improvements in provider performance to a change in how providers are paid.
- It remains to be seen how these innovations can make contributions to improving health care quality or efficiency in the long-run.

This report has identified a number of recommendations for better ways to pay for health care:

Continue innovation to payment systems to reward good outcomes of care

- Payers should continue to explore payment innovations in their settings and better align payment systems with health policy objectives, and providers should be rewarded for what they deliver – not simply what they can do.
- All innovative provider payment models – add-on payments, bundled payments and population-based payments – should encourage further gathering of data (included linkages of data across different datasets) to improve knowledge about the links between health care activities and outcomes.
- Efforts to clarify health policy objectives and encourage more informed dialogue between purchasers and providers need to be an important element of payment innovation reforms.

Design payment innovations grounded on scientific evidence and encourage transparency

- Draw on evidence-based guidelines to inform tariffs. Transparent criteria contribute to better adherence to treatment protocols and more standardised care.

- Use transparent criteria to define the patient populations to the payment innovation – for example if it is only applicable to selected patients (e.g. high-risk patients or patients with multi-morbidity).
- Encourage quality targets to be based on best practice guidelines defined by institutions in charge of defining good practices for the payment innovation. Use a wide set of quality measures to make care delivery and performance more transparent for payers particularly for bundled and population-based payments.
- Use digital innovations and IT systems to help generate new evidence, identify high-need patients and facilitate interoperability of IT systems across health providers.

Implement payment innovations through consensus and engagement with stakeholders

- Target stakeholders from the start and keep them engaged.
- Share joint aims and motivation among key stakeholders to achieve buy-in, particularly for mitigating diverging financial interests.
- Reach a consensus among payers and providers on which quality targets to use in the payment reform.
- Make use of existing data and reporting requirements as a good starting point to minimise administrative burden.
- Strike a balance between additional data reporting requirements on quality and outcomes and the associated administrative burden for providers.

Make evaluation of payment innovations an ongoing activity

- Pilot experimentation into the payment policy before being rolled-out on a larger scale.
- Allow for flexibility in the payment reform to adjust policy parameters if incentives do not have the desired effects.
- Embed evaluation into the payment reform to strengthen accountability and transparency of the payment policy.
- Encourage systematic independent evaluation to improve analysis as very often there are no control groups, and observable changes in quality, outcome or efficiency indicators cannot always be unambiguously attributed to changes in the payment scheme.
- Encourage monitoring, evaluation and feedback reporting to providers on a systematic basis as this has shown to encourage provider support and improve care processes.

Notes

1. The "Contrat de l'amélioration des pratiques individuelles" (CAPI) targeting GPs was replaced by the 'Rémuneration sur objectifs de santé publique' (ROSP) in 2012, which also opened the scheme to outpatient specialists.

2. A risk compensation mechanism exists in the German Statutory Health Insurance Scheme taking into account different distributions of age and diseases of the insured among the 140 public health insurers

References

Acerte, B., A. Stafford and P. Stapleton (2011), "Spanish Healthcare Public Private Partnerships: The 'Alzira Model'", *Critical Perspectives on Accounting*, Vol. 22, pp. 533-549.

Addicott, R. and M. Shortell (2014), "How Accountable Are Accountable Care Organizations?", *Health Care Management Review*, Vol. 39, No. 4, pp. 270-278.

American College of Emergency Physicians (2015), "Medicare's Hospital Readmission Reduction Program FAQ", retrieved at: https://www.acep.org/Physician-Resources/Practice-Resources/Administration/Financial-Issues-/-Reimbursement/Medicare-s-Hospital-Readmission-Reduction-Program-FAQ/.

Barnes, A.J. et al. (2014), "Accountable Care Organizations in the USA: Types, Developments and Challenges", *Health Policy*, Vol. 118, pp. 1-7.

Brammli-Greenberg, S. et al (2015), "How Israel Reimburses Hospitals Based on Activity: The Procedure-related Group (PRG) Incremental Reform", Report submitted for the OECD Project on Payment Systems.

Busse, R. (2011), "Payment Systems to Improve Quality, Efficiency, and Care Coordination for Chronically Ill Patients", Presentation at the International Symposium On Health Care Policy, Washington D.C., 8-10 November.

Busse, R and J. Stahl (2014), "Integrated Care Experiences and Outcomes in Germany, the Netherlands, and England", *Health Affairs*, Vol. 33, No. 9, pp. 1549-1558.

Cashin, C. et al. (2014), "Paying for Performance in Health Care: Implications for Health System Performance and Aaccountability", European Observatory on Health Systems and Policies, OECD and L'Assurance Maladie, Open Universtiy Press, Maidenhead.

Commonwealth Fund (2015), *International Profiles of Health Care Systems 2014*, Washington, DC.

De Bruin, S.R. et al. (2012), "Impact of Disease Management Programs on Healthcare Expenditures for Patients with Diabetes, Depression, Heart Failure or Chronic Obstructive Pulmonary Disease: A Systematic Review of the Literature", *Health Policy*, Vol. 101, pp. 105-121.

Delnoij, D., N. Klazinga and I.K. Glasgow (2002), "Integrated Care in an International Perspective", *International Journal of Integrated Care*, Vol. 2, No. 1, pp. 1-4.

Eijkenaar, F. et al. (2013), "Effects of Pay for Performance in Health Care: A Systematic Review of Systematic Reviews", *Health Policy*, Vol. 110, pp. 115-130.

Gershlick, B (2015), "Best Practice Tariffs Case Study", Report submitted for the OECD Project on Payment Systems.

Hildebrandt, H., T. Schulte and B. Stunder (2012), "Triple Aim in Kinzigtal, Germany", *Journal of Integrated Care*, Vol. 20, No. 4, pp. 205-222.

IDF – International Diabetes Federation (2013), *IDF Diabetes Atlas*, 6th Edition, International Diabetes Federation, Brussels, http://www.idf.org/diabetesatlas/previouseditions.

IRDES – Insitut de recherche et documentation en économie de la santé (2014a), "L'évaluation de la performance des maisons, pôles et centres de santé dans le cadre des Expérimentations des nouveaux modes de rémunération (ENMR) sur la période 2009-2012", *Les Rapports de L'IRDES*, No. 559, December.

IRDES (2014b), "Les formes du regroupement pluriprofessional en soins de premier recours", *Questions d'économie de la santé*, No. 201, September.

Kocot, S.L. et al. (2014), "A More Complete Picture of Pioneer ACO Result", Brooking Institute, available at http://www.brookings.edu/blogs/up-front/posts/2014/10/09-pioneer-aco-results-mcclellan#recent_rr/.

Léger, P.T. (2008), "Physician Payment Mechanisms", in M. Lu and E. Jonsson (eds.), *Financing Health Care: New Ideas for a Changing Society*, Wiley-VCH Verlag GmbH & Co. KGaA, Weinheim, Germany.

McWilliams, J.M. et al. (2014), "Changes in Patients' Experiences in Medicare Accountable Care Organizations", *New England Journal of Medicine*, Vol. 371, No. 18, pp. 1715-1724.

Milstein, R. and C.R. Blankart (2014), "Integrated Care in Germany", Report submitted for the OECD Project on Payment Systems, http://www.oecd.org/health/paying-providers.htm.

Ministère des Affaires Sociales, de la Santé et des Droits des Femmes (2015), "Communiqué de Presse – 20 février 2015", Paris, http://www.social-sante.gouv.fr/IMG/pdf/03_09_13_CP_PTMG.pdf.

Mnich, E. et al. (2013), "Outcome Evaluation of a Health Promotion Among the Elderly", *Gesundheitswesen*, Vol. 75, No. 02, pp. e05-e10.

Nolte, E. and C. Knai (2014), "Approaches to Chronic Disease Management in Europe", in E. Nolte, C. Knai and R.B. Saltman (eds.), "Assessing Chronic Disease Management in European Health Systems – Concepts and Approaches", European Observatory Study Series 37, World Health Organization.

Nolte, E. and M. McKee (2008), *Caring for People with Chronic Conditions: A Health System Perspective*, Open University Press, Maidenhead.

Norwegian Directorate of Health (2014), "Quality Based Financing in Norway", Report submitted for the OECD Project on Payment Systems.

Nuffield Trust (2012), "Reforming Payment for Health Care in Europe to Achieve Better Value", Research Report, London.

OECD (2014), "Paying Providers for Health Care. Results of the 2012 Health Systems Characteristics Survey", data files at http://www.oecd.org/els/health-systems/paying-providers.htm.

OECD (2012), "Ageing, Non-communicable Diseases (NCDs) and Emerging Models of Care", OECD Fast-track Paper.

Or, Z. and U. Häkinnen (2011), "DRGs and Quality: For Better or Worse?", in R. Busse et al. (eds.), *Diagnosis-Related Groups in Europe – Moving Towards Transparency, Efficiency and Quality in Hospitals*, Open University Press.

Robinson, J.C. (2001), "Theory and Practice in the Design of Physician Payment Incentives", *Milbank Quarterly*, Vol. 79, pp. 149-177.

Shortell, S.M., R.P. Gillies and D.A. Anderson (1994), "The New World of Managed Care: Creating Organized Delivery Systems", *Health Affairs*, Vol. 13, No. 5, p. 46.

Shortell, S.M. et al. (2014), "Accountable Care Organisations in the United States and England: Testing, Evaluation and Learning What Works", The King's Fund.

Simoens, S. and A. Scott (1999), "Towards a Definition and Taxonomy of Integration in Primary Care", University of Aberdeen.

Song, Z.; et al. (2014), "Changes in Health Spending and Quality 4 Years into Global Payment", *New England Journal of Medicine*, Vol. 371, No. 18, pp. 1704-1714.

Struijs, J.N. et al. (2012a), "Three Years of Bundled Payment for Diabetes Care in the Netherlands – Impact on Health Care Delivery Process and the Quality of Care", National Institute for Public Health and the Environment (RIVM), Bilthoven.

Struijs, J.N. et al. (2012b), "Effects of Bundled Payment on Curative Health Care Costs in the Netherlands – An Analysis for Diabetes Care and Vascular Risk Management Based on Nationwide Claim Data, 2007-2010", National Institute for Public Health and the Environment (RIVM), Bilthoven.

Vlaanderen, F.P. et al. (2015), "The Dutch Outcome-based Payment Model of ParkinsonNet: A Case Study", Report submitted for the OECD Project on Payment Systems.

Werblow, A. and A. Karmann (2012), "Evaluation des integrierten Versorgungsvertrages über die Versorgung kardiovaskuulär erkrankter Versicherter (CARDIO-Integral) der AOK Plus" [Evaluation of the integrated care programme on the delivery of care to enrollees with cardiovascular diseases], Dresden.

White House (2014), "Historically Slow Growth in Health Spending Continued in 2013, and Data Show Underlying Slow Cost Growth Is Continuing".

Chapter 1

Reforming traditional health care provider payments

This chapter presents an overview of the predominant payment systems used in OECD countries to pay health care providers, notably in primary care, outpatient specialist care and hospital settings. These payment methods include fee-for-service (FFS), capitation, global budgets and salary and more recently, payment per case/diagnosis related groups in the hospital setting. Each payment method generates incentives, likely to affect provider behaviour and the predominant payment systems do not always provide the right incentives and tend to encourage volume of services and increases in health spending. These "traditional" ways of paying providers are often not well adapted to contemporary health system challenges, for instance the need to increase co-ordination of care, or provide high quality care for chronic diseases. While some OECD countries have begun to reform their traditional payments, others have introduced payment innovations that are more closely tied to key health system objectives of efficiency and quality of care.

The statistical data for Israel are supplied by and under the responsibility of the relevant Israeli authorities. The use of such data by the OECD is without prejudice to the status of the Golan Heights, East Jerusalem and Israeli settlements in the West Bank under the terms of international law.

1.1. Overview

Across OECD health systems a variety of policy levers are used to help meet health system objectives. One such important lever is the way health care providers are paid for services they deliver. Most often, health care providers are paid in the same way they always have been, using the traditional, dominant payment methods common across OECD health systems. However, these ways of paying providers – through fee-for-service (FFS), capitation, salary, global budget or more recently diagnosis-related groups (DRG) – are often poorly aligned with health system priorities. Rather than giving incentives to providers to improve quality, or deliver care more efficiently, these "traditional" payment methods come with a host of built-in incentives for unwanted consequences, for instance over-provision of services or inattention to clinical need.

Traditional payment systems are particularly challenged by the shift in care needs many health systems in OECD countries are currently confronted with. Ageing societies and changes in life styles such as unhealthy diet and physical inactivity have led to a rise in the prevalence of chronic conditions. In addition, more and more patients now suffer from multiple morbidities. New care models centered around the patient have been developed to address the needs of those requiring the co-ordination of activities among different health providers working in various settings. Traditionally, payment systems do little to support these new care models as health service provision is predominantly financed in a "silo" way. This implies a strict separation in the financing of the various health providers with few incentives for co-operation across sectors. Frequently, this contributes to fragmentation of care with poor patient experience and health outcome.

This chapter provides an overview of the traditional payment approaches used in OECD health systems, their use in different parts of health systems, and details some of their shortcomings leading to the question of why there is a need to reform health care provider payment systems. It then goes on to present some recent trends in select OECD countries, where traditional payment mechanisms like FFS or DRGs have been adapted to better align payment objectives with health system objectives. Finally, the chapter presents recent thinking about ways of transforming traditional payment systems, to the more radical and innovative approaches to payment reform in the subsequent chapters.

1.2. Why reform provider payment?

How providers are paid is one of the key policy levers that countries have to drive health system performance. Yet, payment systems too often do not pay for improvements in health outcomes, but rather reward providers for increased outputs. Likewise, budget constraints and the structure of the health care provider market in particular countries influence the extent to which payment systems encourage increased productivity or quality. Recent policy development and research have focussed on the idea that payment systems should evolve towards paying providers for the value they add to a patient's health instead of paying for inputs or providers' activities.

Overall, payment systems in many OECD countries have evolved beyond simple FFS and global or input-based budgets. Primary care payments have become more heterogeneous as countries seek to combine various elements of payments with differing intensities in out-patient care. FFS has been increasingly supplemented by additional payments to encourage gate keeping and co-ordination of care. Countries using capitation and budgets have added elements to drive quality or increase productivity. In hospitals, there has been a shift to financing on the basis of DRGs (Box 1.1), primarily to encourage providers to increase efficiency by reducing their production costs per case. Beyond these broad trends, there has been increasing experimentation with new ways of paying providers.

Box 1.1. Diagnosis-related groups in OECD health systems

Payment per case based on diagnosis-related groups (DRG) were first implemented in the 1980s in the United States to finance inpatient services to address the shortcomings of previous dominant modes of payment such as FFS and prospective global budgets. Since then, hospital payment via DRG has become increasingly popular among OECD countries and beyond. DRGs are also increasingly used in low- and middle-income countries and the Asia-Pacific region.

Although DRG has frequently become synonymous with a mode of payment, it is first and foremost a patient classification system. The aim of this classification system is the grouping of patients with similar conditions requiring similar intensity of treatment into the same category. Typically, patients are allocated to one DRG based on their diagnoses and the procedures performed. In many DRG systems, severity is also taken into account when determining a DRG group. Frequently, each DRG group is associated with a relative weighting reflecting the cost of treatment clustered in this group against a benchmark group. Summing up the relative weights per patient treated in a given hospital over a time period defines the case-mix. Comparing the case-mix per hospital or region allows for an assessment of where the more severely affected, cost-intensive patients are treated. With few exceptions, most OECD countries have used existing DRG classifications and adapted them to their country-specific circumstances.

In countries where DRGs are used as a payment system, the relative weights per DRG are multiplied by a nominal base rate – a monetary conversion rate – to define the amount of money a hospital receives from the payer for the treatment of a patient. The nominal base rate can differ between regions and even between hospitals. The relative weights per DRG are calculated by countries using national cost-accounting data from all or a subset of hospitals, except where countries decided to import cost weights from other countries with the assumption that relative costs between the same patient groups would not differ between countries (Siok Swann et al., 2011). The average costs across hospitals (or a sub-set) are used as the basis of the calculation. Alternatively, in some health systems, DRGs are directly translated into a monetary tariff without the use of relative weighting.

DRG tariffs are frequently adjusted in case of outliers and, in many cases, hospitals can receive additional payments for costs which are not factored in a DRG tariff such as expensive medication or capital costs. A central characteristic of a DRG tariff is that it is known prospectively and independent of the length of stay of a patient. Hence, hospitals have a strong incentive to provide care efficiently and to discharge the patient as soon as possible after recovery.

Source: Kobel et al. (2011); Siok Swan et al. (2011); Mathauer and Wittenbecher (2012); Mathauer and Wittenbecher (2013); Kwon and Shon (2015).

In this context, it is worthwhile to take stock of the profile of payment systems in the OECD and highlight promising innovations that could shed light on how provider payments might evolve in the next ten years, and beyond.

The discussion in this publication focusses on financial incentives for providers and does not explore other forms of incentives of health professionals which also influence health system performance. Non-financial health system levers include performance feedback or public reporting of health professionals' performance to drive quality improvements and can be used as an element to accompany payment reforms or implemented independently (see for example *OECD Health Care Quality Review* series).

Like other economic actors, health providers can be expected to respond to financial incentives, however, they are not exclusively motivated by monetary considerations. Economic actors are also intrinsically motivated (Gneezy et al., 2011). They care about their reputation, can get satisfaction out of an activity they enjoy doing and may also be motivated by altruistic motives. This is important to bear in mind when discussing whether – paradoxically – financial incentives may have negative consequences for performance by crowding out intrinsic motivation. This phenomenon has been observed in particular in cases where incentives were targeted at individuals to encourage contributions to public goods (Gneezy et al., 2011). With regards to health care provision this hypothesis suggests that economic incentives to encourage certain activities, for example, making bonus payments dependent on meeting quality objectives, could potentially backfire and lead to worse health outcomes. Health professionals may be demotivated by limitations in their clinical autonomy. Monetary incentives may also damage the self-esteem of doctors who perceive financial rewards for quality as a "de-valuation" of their professional code (Marshall and Harrison, 2005). Whether this translates into worse health care performance is unknown. Analysing impact of financial incentives in the P4P programme in the United Kingdom, McDonald et al. (2007) find no reduction in intrinsic motivation of general practitioners (GPs).

1.3. Traditional provider payment systems and misaligned incentives

Traditional payment methods defined

In OECD countries, the most commonly used approaches to pay health care providers are payment i) per consultation/procedure (FFS), ii) per registered patient (capitation), iii) for services carried out over a defined period of time (e.g. salary, global budget), and iv) payment per case (e.g. diagnosis-related groups). Some of the main features distinguishing these methods are whether payments are defined before health care delivery (prospective) or after (retrospective) and the extent to which different services are bundled in a single tariff (Table 1.1).

Table 1.1. An overview of traditional payment methods in health care systems

Payment method	Description	Setting	Degree of bundling
Fee-for-service (FFS)	Retrospective activity-based payment: billing of individual services and patient contacts	Predominant mode of payment for GPs and for outpatient specialist services	unbundled
Payment per case (diagnosis-related groups)	Prospective activity-based payment per patient, patient classified into groups based on diagnoses and resource use	Payment for hospital inpatient cases in many countries	↕
Capitation	Prospective lump-sum payment per enrolled patient covering a range of services	Mode of payment for GPs in a number of countries	
Global budget	Prospective lump-sum payment covering a range of services independent of actual volume provided	Payment for public hospitals in a number of countries	bundled

Note: The predominant method of payment was determined by countries based on its share of total spending, number of contacts or number of providers (*OECD Health Systems Characteristics Survey 2012*).

Source: Adapted from Charlesworth et al. (2012).

FFS is the most unbundled payment as every activity performed under this scheme can be billed separately. Global budgets on the other hand represent the most bundled form of payment with a lump sum covering a range of services independent of actual volume provided. Another important characteristic of payment mechanisms refers to the extent health providers are exposed to the financial risk of service provision (Figure 1.1).

Figure 1.1. Exposure to financial risk for payers and providers

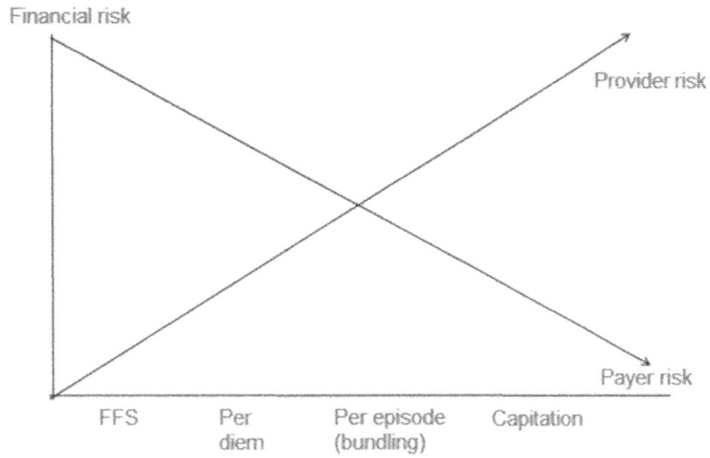

Source: Adapted from Jegers et al. (2002).

From the perspective of a general practitioner, FFS and capitation are at the opposing ends of the risk spectrum. FFS schemes bear no financial risk to the provider while the payer is exposed to all risk. This means the payer encounters the risk of covering all costs for service provision in case the patient requires more health care than envisaged. Conversely, under capitation schemes it is the provider who is exposed to most risk as he will only receive one payment but may have to face high number of visits per patient without additional payments.

Other types of "traditional" payment such as line-item budgets or per diem payments are still marginally used in OECD health systems, but have been mostly phased out from systems because of the negative incentives associated with them. Indeed, payment using per diems or "bed days" is widely understood to incentivise excessively long lengths of stay in inpatient settings, presenting a greater financial burden to the system with no therapeutic benefit to the patient. Per diem payments still remain more common in some settings where DRG implementation has been particularly challenging, notably mental health care (OECD, 2014a) and long-term care.

Depending on the health systems context and organisation, payments are made out to individuals or various types of entities for the provision of specific types of service. Primary care services could be provided by a self-employed general practitioner, by a small practice combining several health professionals, or a multi-disciplinary clinic. The provider of specialist or tertiary services is often a hospital, but could also be an independently practicing specialist. If a payment is made out to an entity, it will in turn compensate the health professionals. Incentives created by the payment to the institution and to actual provider can conflict.

Traditional and widely used provider payment mechanisms often bring unwanted incentives

There is little doubt that the overwhelming majority of health providers care about the well-being of their patients and are motivated by improving their health status, but it is generally acknowledged that they also respond to financial incentives (McGuire, 2000; Chandra et al., 2012). Hence, health providers adjust their clinical decisions according to the way they are paid. This can incentivise health providers to an inefficient over- or under-provision of medical services. The impact of traditional payment systems on provider behaviour has been shown theoretically as well as empirically (Gosden et al., 2000; Street et al., 2011; Iverson, 2015; or Murakami and Lorenzoni, 2015). All modes of payment have strengths and weaknesses when it comes to meeting policy objectives and in their "pure" form; that is, as standalone payment methods without additional forms of blended payments or adjustments, traditional modes of payment face particular challenges to meet some of today's health system priorities. Table 1.2 displays the expected effects of FFS, capitation, global budget and case-based payment (diagnosis-related groups) on some key dimensions of health system performance.

Table 1.2. Expected impact of payment systems on dimensions of health system performance

Payment method	Activity		Expenditure control	Technical efficiency	Quality
	Number of cases	Number of services/case			
Fee-for-service	↑	↑	↓	0	0
DRG-based payment	↑	↓	0	↑	0
Global budget	↓	↓	↑	0	0
Capitation	↑	↓	↑	↑	0

Note: Legend: ↑ increase; ↓ decrease; 0 neutral or unclear.

Source: Adapted from Geissler et al. (2011).

Table 1.3 provides a summary of some expected advantages and some possible unintended consequences of traditional payment systems in their pure form. The impact of payment systems also depend in part on the setting in which they are used and other policy measures that can affect care delivery and utilisation.

Table 1.3. Theoretical advantages and disadvantages of traditional payment systems

	FFS	Capitation	Global budget	DRG
Reasons to implement	• Better compliance to guidelines with required number of visits • Quicker uptake of innovative activities • Less risk selection issues • Improving access • Transparency	• Cost control • Low transaction costs • Higher focus on preventive activities	• Cost control • Low transaction cost	• Increasing activity when replacing global budget • Decreasing activity when replacing FFS • Increased technical efficiency • Reduction in average length of stay • Equity • Reduction in waiting time • Transparency
Possible unintended consequences	• High clinical activity (number of visits and services per patients) • Associated with higher costs • High transaction costs	• Increase in number of patients • Possible skimping of care (fewer visits per patient and less activity per patient) • Quicker referrals to other providers • Possible risk selection	• Rationing of services with increased waiting time • Possible skimping of care (fewer visits per patient and less activity per patient) • Budget allocation may be less transparent	• Hospitals trying to attract additional patients • Focus on more profitable activities • Associated with higher total costs • High transaction costs • Early discharges • Upcoding • Possible risk selection

Source: Authors' compilation.

Fee-for-service can lead to volume and cost inflation

FFS encourages the provision of high volumes of services. Theoretically, providers have the incentive to increase the number of patients or patient visits and also the number of services performed per patient if no additional activity-limiting measures are in place. This hypothesis was confirmed in a number of studies. For example, a systematic review of studies by Gosden et al. (2000) concluded that in primary care the number of visits was higher under a FFS scheme compared to capitation or for salaried physicians. The same result was found by Peckham and Glousia (2014). In Norway, prior to 2001, primary care physicians paid through a mix of FFS and block grant were found to have a higher number of visits than their salaried colleagues (Sorensen and Grytten, 2003). Similar results are found in Canada (Dumont et al., 2008; Kantarevic and Kralj, 2013). One study in the province of Ontario found that physicians under FFS relative to other payment schemes saw more patients (Devlin and Sarma, 2008). A cross-sectional survey of a sample of physicians in the United States found that physicians paid by capitation were more likely to be conservative in the use of resources than physicians paid using FFS (Shen et al., 2004). If no volume caps are in place, FFS can lead to inefficient over-provision of services and thus, rising costs.

Capitation and global budget impose limits on cost and volume

Capitation or global budgets help to control costs as they do not encourage increasing volumes of services, but they come with other challenges. In the case of capitation, providers are encouraged to increase the number of enrolled patients (within the bounds of any cap on patient numbers), but also to reduce the number of services provided to each of them. This can increase technical efficiency in service provision as it encourages providers to make better use of available resources. Yet, capitation payments are associated with a level of clinical activity below patient preferences making them not socially optimal (Iverson, 2015).

The incentives for providers paid via global budgets and salaried physicians are similar. Providers receiving a global budget and salaried professionals are both encouraged to provide fewer services than under FFS. Unlike capitation, global budgets do not motivate physicians to increase the number of patients. Global budgets are not associated with an efficient use of resources if they are based on historic spending or inputs used. Global budgets and salaries are effective in putting a cap on provider costs, but this may in turn lead to rationing of services and extended waiting times.

Quality objectives not easily met by traditional payment systems

Incentives to improve the quality of care are not inherent in FFS, capitation and global budget (salaries) and their effects on quality are not clear. In theory, capitation payments should encourage health providers to engage patients in preventive activities to avoid more costly treatment later. But if limited to the primary care sector, capitation payments can incentivise GPs to refer patients early to less appropriate care settings. This may translate in reduced quality and negative patient experience.

FFS schemes can encourage GPs to comply with guidelines in case these foresee a recommended number of visits. This finding was reported by Gosden et al. (2000) comparing the compliance to guidelines for GPs paid by FFS to those paid under capitation or salaried physicians. Gosden et al. (2000) also found fewer referrals and more continuity of care for physicians paid for by FFS. Sorbero et al. (2003) find that chronic patients are less likely to switch primary care physicians when their physician is paid by FFS than under capitation. This could be an indication of better care quality, at least in terms of patient experience. Analysing physician's behaviour under managed care contracts in the United States, Melichar (2009) finds that physicians spend less time with those patients for whom they receive a capitation than with those patients for whom they are paid for differently. Whether this is due to skimping of care for capitated patients or due to a reduction of unnecessary services that do not affect health outcomes – and thus improving efficiency – is not clear. In a systematic review of the impact of payment systems in dental care, Brocklehurst et al. (2013) found evidence that dentists under capitation provide more advice on prevention, but had less frequent appointments with their patients and restored their teeth at later stages of the disease process than dentists paid under alternative schemes. However, to what extent physicians under FFS are engaging in preventive activity will also depend on the relative prices in the fee schedule. In the case of the United States, the National Commission on Physician Payment reform recommended to increase the fees for preventive activities and other undervalued services at the expense of procedural diagnosis to address a perceived under-provision of specific services (Schroeder and Frist, 2013).

FFS with no apparent access problem

FFS is a relatively transparent way of paying providers for listed services and can be adapted relatively easy to changes in care provision, such as the addition of a new pharmaceutical, service or procedure. From an administrative point of view, billing each activity per patient is typically more burdensome for providers with higher transaction costs than other more bundled modes of payment, such as capitation or global budgets.

Typically, there are few issues with access to care under a FFS system. Physicians have no reason to select or cherry-pick patients if they are rewarded for all services they provide. This is different under capitation or global budget. If capitated payments are not risk-adjusted, providers will try to select positive risks by enrolling predominantly healthy patients. Potentially, this presents a real barrier to access for chronic patients. Under global budgets cherry-picking can also be an issue, as well as rationing of services and increased waiting times.

Overall, a number of authors advocate the use of blended payment, for example a mix of FFS and capitation in primary care (Iverson, 2015) to achieve the socially optimal volume of services. While many countries experiment with blended forms of payment in primary care, there is no clear evidence on the optimal blend of payment schemes (Peckham and Glousia, 2014; Rudoler et al., 2015).

Payment per case focusses on efficiency

In the hospital sector, payment per case such as for diagnosis-related groups (DRG) can have mixed incentives, depending on the design and implementation in a payment system. A prime motivation behind the implementation is to improve the efficient use of hospital resources. Receiving a single tariff per patient, hospitals will be eager to reduce their production costs to generate profits.

Reviewing a wide range of studies, Street et al. (2011) conclude that in the majority of cases, the introduction of DRG systems led to higher total costs, whereas the growth in total costs slowed down after the introduction of DRG in the United States. Summarising recent evidence in OECD countries, Murakami and Lorenzoni (2015) report mixed evidence with regards to a decrease of costs per discharge.

A reduction of the average length of stay after the implementation of DRG-based payments – at least initially – is generally found in OECD countries and beyond (Moreno-

Serra and Wagstaff, 2010; Street et al., 2011; Murakami and Lorenzoni, 2015). The impact on overall activity and costs is less clear. Depending on the mode of payment DRG payments were seeking to replace, this change has led to an increase (Australia, Denmark, England, France, Germany, Norway, and Spain) or a decrease (United States) in hospital activity (Street et al., 2011; Schreyögg et al., 2014). This suggests that hospitalisation volumes increase in countries where case-based payments replace general budgets or where DRG are used to set hospital budgets. However, analysing data from Central and Eastern European countries and Central Asia, Moreno-Serra and Wagstaff (2010) find no increase in hospital admission for countries that replaced historical budgets with case-based payment. Activity tends to decrease where DRG replace cost-based reimbursement schemes such as FFS.

The possible rise in hospital activity after introduction of case-based payment in a number of OECD countries may be systematic. There is some evidence that hospitals bring up activity in domains which are most profitable for hospitals (Busse et al., 2011). This is the case for those clinical areas where the DRG tariffs based on average hospital costs lie above the cost of service provision for a particular hospital. There is also some evidence of spill-over effects to other sectors as a consequence of the introduction of case-based payment. This can refer to a general increase in discharges to post-acute facilities as concluded by Palmer et al. (2014) in a systematic review of recent evidence from ten OECD countries, or to shifts from inpatient to day care or outpatient settings (Street et al., 2011). Hence, the introduction of DRG can influence total hospitals costs as well as health spending in general, but whether the effect is positive or negative will also depend on the payment system case-based payment is seeking to replace. Street et al. (2011) conclude that in the majority of cases the introduction of DRG systems has led to higher total costs whereas total cost growth was slowed down after introduction of DRG in the United States. Wagstaff and Moreno (2010), too, find overall increased health spending after the introduction of case-based payment.

The reduction of waiting times is also frequently named as an objective when introducing case-based payment in hospitals. This has been achieved for example in Sweden (Serden, 2011). However, causality may be difficult to establish if the introduction of case-based payment is accompanied with other initiatives to bring down waiting times, as seen in England (Appleby et al., 2012).

Quality effects are less clear for payment per case

The impact of the introduction of DRGs on quality is unclear. DRGs make payment transparent, which should lead to a greater standardisation of care and improved comparability (Or and Häkkinen, 2011). Striving to find efficiency gains, DRG implementation may also lead to a faster adoption of new technology. Confronted with a single tariff, hospitals in a competitive environment may start to compete for patients by driving up quality. On the other hand, in their quest to achieve efficiency gains, hospitals may skimp on care and discharge patients too early if paid under a DRG regime. Supplementing DRGs with additional payments for outliers, high cost input or the adoption of new technology can be a policy measure to address issues around under-treatment or risk selection by hospitals (Appleby et al., 2012).

Summarising the existing studies, Or and Häkkinen (2011) report that there is evidence in the United States that the implementation of DRG has led to improvements in organisational efficiency and quality of care in some areas by developing home-based care and ambulatory care options. However, they also found some limited evidence for increased readmission and mortalities in the United States. They found no confirmation of these negative effects in Europe. The review of Palmer et al. (2014) suggests a possible increase in readmission but no consistent impact on mortality in acute or post-acute care. Summarising recent evidence, Murakami and Lorenzoni (2015) could not observe any general detrimental impact on quality of care after the introduction of case-based payment, but highlight that existing evidence is very limited.

Administrative burden with DRGs

DRG payments are administratively very complex and hospitals have incentives to "up-code" their patients to overstate the severity of a case to trigger higher payments. Up-coding was identified as a concern in France, for example, where outpatient cases were wrongly recorded as day cases instead of outpatient care (Or and Häkkinen, 2011). Typically, up-coding can be addressed by better auditing and systematic control of hospital billing.

Wider health system effects

There may also be a possible interaction between payment of the institution and payment of health professionals working within the institution. In some cases, payment schemes for the institution delivering care and professionals working in this institution may bear conflicting incentives, for instance a hospital that receives case-based payments (volume incentives) with salaried physicians (no volume incentives) but little is known of any potential overall effect.

In general, the strengths and weaknesses of traditional payment systems in their "pure" form led countries to respond in three ways: i) blending payment methods to counterbalance their individual shortcomings; ii) adapting traditional modes of payment in an intelligent way; iii) developing new innovative ways to pay providers.

1.4. The use of blended payment methods across health care settings and recent trends

Despite their inherent challenges, traditional payment methods remain the main mode of paying providers in OECD countries. They are used to varying extents in OECD health systems, and their implementation or ongoing use is usually determined by the care setting, the type of provider and other health system characteristics.

Clear patterns in the way traditional payment methods are used can be observed across OECD health systems. Table 1.4 summarises the main modes of payment by countries' key purchasers in the year 2012. Notably, capitation is used exclusively in primary care, while FFS is common for both primary and outpatient specialist care. In primary care, and to a slightly lesser extent in outpatient specialist care, many countries employ more than one traditional payment mechanism simultaneously. Compared to the results of the 2008 OECD Health Systems Characteristics Survey, the number of countries that use a mix of payment systems for primary care and outpatient specialist care appears to be growing (Paris et al., 2010). In inpatient care, too, most countries apply a mix of payment schemes. For service provision in public hospitals DRGs and global budgets are the most commonly used main methods of payment. The use of multiple payment forms for given care setting can mean either a blending of payments (i.e. a GP practice which is paid through a combination of FFS and P4P) or different providers paid in different ways (i.e. some primary care clinics paid by capitation, while others are paid with FFS). Finally it can mean that different key payers use different payment methods for the same type of service.

Table 1.4. Use of traditional forms of provider payment by care setting in OECD countries

	Provider payment		
	Primary care	Outpatient specialist care	Inpatient[1]
Australia	FFS/P4P	FFS	DRG
Austria	FFS	FFS	DRG
Belgium	CAP/FFS	FFS	Global budget
Canada	CAP/FFS/P4P	FFS/Global Budget/Other	Global budget
Chile	CAP/FFS	FFS/Global Budget	Procedure service
Czech Republic	CAP/FFS/P4P	FFS	DRG
Denmark	CAP/FFS	Other	Global budget
Estonia	CAP/FFS/P4P/Global	FFS	DRG
Finland	Global Budget	FFS	DRG
France	FFS/P4P/Other	FFS/P4P/Other	DRG
Germany	FFS	FFS	DRG
Greece	FFS	FFS	DRG
Hungary	CAP/P4P/Global Bud	FFS	DRG
Iceland	Global Budget	FFS	Global budget
Ireland	CAP/FFS	Global Budget	Global budget
Israel	CAP/Global Budget	Global Budget	Procedure service
Italy	CAP	FFS/Global Budget	Global budget
Japan[2]	FFS	FFS	DRG/Procedure service
Korea[3]	FFS/P4P	FFS/P4P	Procedure service
Luxembourg	FFS	FFS	Global budget
Mexico	CAP/Global Budget	FFS/Global Budget	Global budget
Netherlands	CAP/FFS/P4P/Global	FFS/P4P	DRG
New Zealand	CAP/FFS/P4P	Global Budget	Global budget
Norway	CAP/FFS	FFS/Global Budget/Other	Global budget
Poland	CAP	Other	DRG
Portugal	CAP/P4P/Global Bud	P4P/Global Budget	Global budget
Slovak Republic	CAP/FFS	FFS	Procedure service
Slovenia	CAP/FFS	FFS	DRG
Spain	CAP/P4P	FFS/Global Budget	Line-item remuneration
Sweden	CAP/FFS/P4P	FFS/P4P/Global Budget	Global budget
Switzerland	CAP/FFS	FFS	DRG
Turkey	CAP/P4P	Global Budget	Global budget
United Kingdom	CAP/FFS/P4P/Other	P4P/Global Budget/Other	DRG
United States[4]	CAP/FFS/P4P/Other	FFS/P4P/Global Budget	DRG

Note: CAP refers to capitation; FFS refers to fee-for-service; P4P refers to pay for performance. The predominant method of payment presented was determined by countries based on its share of total spending, number of contacts or number of providers. Table 1.4 displays all main modes of payment for primary care and outpatient care by key purchasers but only the most important method to pay public hospitals in inpatient care.

1. Refers to public hospitals (only the main mode of payment identified).

2. No predominant mode of payment exists for inpatient care services in public hospitals in Japan.

3. It is difficult to distinguish between primary care and outpatient specialist care in Korea.

4. Information on inpatient payment refers to the Medicare programme.

Source: OECD Health Systems Characteristics Survey 2012 and OECD Secretariat's estimates.

In primary care, blended forms of payment are used in 25 out of 34 OECD countries. Only nine countries use a single payment form for primary care (capitation, FFS or global budget). All other countries report that at least two forms of payment are used for primary care, either with different payment mechanisms applied to different primary care providers, or individual providers being paid through a blended mix of payment types. The increasingly blended forms of payment in primary care likely indicate a shift towards combining different elements of payments as incentives to meet more specific health policy objectives, or to balance the negative and positive incentives of different payment mechanisms. In Denmark, for example, GPs receive roughly one third of their income from capitation and the remaining from FFS. Service paid via FFS includes after-hours consultations, phone consultations and home visits (Olejaz et al., 2012). In France, the vast majority of income of primary care physicians stems from FFS but additional annual capitated payments for patients with long-term conditions (*"affection de longue durée"*) and bonus payments for meeting pre-defined quality targets are also possible. These pay-for-performance (P4P) elements complement traditional payment modes in primary care in 14 countries (see Chapter 2).

The predominant payment method for outpatient specialist care is FFS, used in 26 out of 34 countries. A much smaller variety of payment types are used within individual countries' outpatient specialist care sector than in the primary care sector. Nevertheless some countries such as Sweden and the United Kingdom have incorporated global budgets for outpatient specialist care along with combinations of P4P. Canada, Norway, Sweden, the United Kingdom and the United States use three main forms of payment for outpatient specialist care.

In the acute inpatient sector, 16 out of 34 countries use case-based funding such as DRG payments as the main method to pay public hospitals. Payment per case is typically associated with hospitals, mainly for inpatient curative treatment but increasingly for day cases, outpatient or rehabilitative treatment. It can be considered as a bundled payment as it combines in a single tariff the payment of a range of services provided during the patient's stay. In about a dozen OECD countries, global budgets are the predominant mode of payment for hospital services. Less common is the use of line-item budgets and payment by procedure as the main form to pay public hospitals.

Some differences in the use of payment mechanisms can be observed between health systems with residence-based health coverage (e.g. the National Health Service in England) and those where coverage is based on contributory payments (e.g. Statutory Health Insurance in Germany). There appears to be a stronger tendency towards DRG-type payments in countries with contributory coverage, while in residence-based coverage systems, there appears to be a tendency towards broader forms of payment for inpatient services in public hospitals (e.g. global budget), though DRG-type payments are also used (Australia, Finland, United Kingdom). Even in systems that predominantly use global budgets to pay public hospitals, DRGs may still exist. In some cases, countries use DRGs as a patient classification tool to allocate budgets rather than explicitly for payment.

These differences in payment between contributory-based and residence-based health systems may in part be related to some of the main financing dimensions of health systems. Countries with contributory-based coverage provided by health insurers may have a more explicit benefit basket where each service has an associated tariff. Differences can also be related to the way services are purchased in health systems. In countries with contributory-based coverage, there typically exists a clear split between purchaser and provider. Here, billing health insurers for the provided services via DRG can be more transparent than negotiating a global budget. On the other hand, in health systems with residence-based coverage, the provider and purchaser of hospital services can be identical (e.g. the Health

Service Executive in Ireland). In these cases, allocating global budgets may be administratively simpler than billing each inpatient case.

Overall, the vast majority of OECD countries use mixed modes to pay for inpatient care in hospitals (Paris et al., 2010). This can mean a combination of DRG and global budgets but also include FFS payments for certain procedures, per-diem rates or line-item payment. An ongoing trend, however, seems to be the increasing interest to implement case-based payment systems.

In Ireland, for example, the implementation of DRG (also called activity-based funding) as a mode of payment is a central element of a more substantial health system reform shifting population coverage from residence-based entitlement towards universal health insurance (UHI)[1] provided by multiple, competing insurers (Department of Health, 2012). Until 2013 hospitals in Ireland were paid for by block grants with some retrospective adjustments for case-mix irrespective of their actual activity. The move towards activity-based funding is to ensure a fairer system of resource allocation where hospitals are encouraged to provide high quality health care, to improve efficiency and increase transparency in the provision of hospital services (Department of Health, 2013).

Greece started using DRGs as part of a large public sector reform which followed the financial and economic crisis. In the health sector, Greece committed to a series of measures to keep public health spending below 6% of GDP, including the modernising management and accounting systems of the hospital sector (European Commission, 2012). Before 2011, public Greek hospitals had fixed budgets covering operational costs and investments but were paid retrospectively for the services they delivered, with little incentive to stay within budget (Economou, 2015). In 2011, Greece began to work on the implementation of a DRG system adapted to the Greek context based on the German DRG system. The main objectives of the introduction of DRG were a reduction of operational expenditures with a specific focus on controlling prices of medical products and services and pharmaceutical consumption; accelerating the invoicing procedure and revenue collection; reducing annual hospital deficits; and balancing expenditure (Polyzos et al., 2013).

In Korea, the move towards case-based payment was more gradual and had to be adapted, mainly because of strong provider resistance. A DRG system was adopted in 2002 to replace a FFS system following concerns about rapidly increasing health care costs in the wake of the introduction of universal health care coverage. The introduction of the K-DRG payment system was limited to seven disease categories referring to a total of 78 DRGs (Kwon and Shon, 2015). Although payment under DRG was more generous compared to fee for service, uptake by hospitals was slow. Hospitals feared constraints in clinical autonomy by not rewarding the use of certain technologies and practices, and that the introduction of DRGs would lead to centrally-driven cost control and a deterioration of quality of care (OECD, 2012). Billing using DRGs was made mandatory to all hospitals and clinics in 2013, but limited to seven disease categories (Kwon and Shon, 2015). In 2009, Korea introduced an alternative payment system called the Korean Case Payment System (KCPS) or "new DRG" which responds to some of the criticism of the K-DRG payment system. Payment under the KCPS combines a DRG base payment with FFS and per diem components. The KCPS can be considered as a move towards more bundled hospital payment as it aims to replace a predominant FFS regime. The KCPS is applied to 550 disease categories and covers around 95% of all inpatient DRG groups of the K-DRG system. In 2013, KCPS was used in 40 local government hospitals (Kwon and Shon, 2015).

As in the case of Korea, the shift towards case-based payment in Israel has been gradual but has gained momentum in recent years (Box 1.2).

Box 1.2. Reforming hospital payment in Israel with data constraints

Israel has been moving towards case-based financing in hospitals over the past decade. Payment per case was introduced on a small scale in the 1990s, but the shift towards more activity-based funding has gained momentum in recent years. Historically, per diem payments (to government hospitals) and FFS (to private hospitals) were the dominant modes of payment in the Israeli hospital sector. The use of per diems is somewhat problematic as the current rates are still based on calculations carried out in 1985. The extent to which these per diems still reflect current cost for treatments is unclear, and the disconnect between payments and costs can lead to over- and under-provision of care.

Another issue that led to the payment reform was that public hospitals were facing growing financial deficits. This is partly due to the fact that private hospitals do not provide emergency care and can select low risk patients for treatment, leaving it up to public hospitals to treat the more severe and costly cases.

In 2002, Israel started a reform of hospital payment which aimed to: reimburse public hospitals in a fairer way; reduce inefficiencies caused by the misalignment between prices and costs; strengthen public hospitals while competing with private hospitals; and improve the level of data collection on activity and quality of care. The incremental change in the payment system is part of a broader health reform aimed at shortening waiting times, increasing hospital activity and using hospital resources more efficiently.

Israel adopted a payment system based on procedures because data on diagnosis were rarely available in such a way that enabled the use of DRGs. Patients are clustered into groups (procedure related groups – PRG) according to the main procedures performed in the course of their treatment. The individual PRG prices are the result of an in-depth costing procedure and extensive discussion among stakeholders. To overcome any possible opposition, it was decided from the outset to include the main actors (Ministry of Health, Ministry of Finance, the four health insurers and hospitals) in the payment reform.

The move towards PRGs was designed as a zero sum game, with no additional funding into the hospital system. This had a direct impact on the price setting of the individual PRGs. If prices of PRGs have to be adjusted downward as a result of budget neutrality, they may no longer adequately reflect their costs which may disincentivise hospitals to provide certain procedures. This reform replaced per diem payment for interventional procedures, while for non-interventional procedures per diem payment still applied.

By 2012, 280 PRGs had been defined, accounting for about 50% of all procedures. The objective was to have 500 PRG by 2015. The share of PRG in total public hospital revenues increased from 16% to 23% between 2003 and 2012, while the share of per diem went down from 47% to 39% over the same period with the remaining revenues mainly stemming from FFS for ambulatory and emergency care. PRGs will need to be developed further, notably, as they currently do not take the severity of patients' condition into account.

Likely due to the incremental introduction of PRG payments and involvement of all stakeholders from the outset, the move towards activity-based funding has been widely supported in Israel. In light of possible alternatives such as importing a DRG system, the development of a classification based on procedural information was considered to be the easiest and least costly alternative. It is also believed that the PRG creates incentives for hospitals to promote the use of advanced technology. A key drawback is that non-interventional procedures are still reimbursed on a per diem basis. The current lack of granularity at the PRG level to take into account different levels of severity of patients' conditions could lead to cherry-picking, encouraging hospitals to treat less complex patient cases. Payment based on procedures also incentivises the over-provision of services.

The reform has led to general improvement and harmonisation of data collection in hospitals, and has motivated hospitals to keep better track of their activities. Hospitals now register diagnosis codes (ICD-9) and procedures performed, which was not required under a per diem payment scheme. The method of micro-costing PRGs is currently reviewed to see whether costs for overhead and medical staff are accurately attributed to individual PRGs. The Ministry has also launched some additional initiatives aimed at improving data availability including a national programme to measure quality in hospitals and the collection of data on waiting times in non-profit hospitals.

No systematic evaluation of the reform has yet been carried out. Based on some preliminary data collected over the period of the PRG implementation, the Israeli Ministry of Health concluded that the PRG has generated some efficiency gains. Average length of stay has gone down, particularly in those departments that previously recorded above average length of stay.

Source: Brammli-Greenberg et al. (2016).

More innovative approaches to implement case-based payments going beyond standard DRG implementation and other ways to bundle activities into a single tariff is discussed in Chapter 3.

1.5. Adapting traditional payment to ensure it is fit for purpose in contemporary health systems

Most OECD countries have adapted traditional payment systems to overcome some of the theoretical disadvantages and make better use of them.

In primary care, nearly all OECD countries adjust the capitation payment made to providers for risk factors to disincentivise skimping of care and cherry-picking. Most countries consider more than one risk dimension in their adjustment procedure. In the calculation of capitation payments 18 countries adjust for age followed by gender (nine countries), health status (nine countries) and utilisation of services (five countries). Twelve countries adjust for other risk factors, such as geographical or socioeconomic factors. Only in Belgium, Denmark, Mexico and Norway capitation is not adjusted. But in these countries, capitation is complemented with an additional mode of payment (OECD, 2014b).

In many cases, global budgets these have evolved beyond resource-based or historical budgets. In hospitals, budget allocation is frequently done on the basis of case-mix as measured via DRGs. This is true, for example, in Portugal (where the case mix weight is around 50% of the total hospital budget) and in some Swedish regions. In addition to making budget setting more transparent, this can also help to benchmark hospitals and incentivise the efficient use of hospital resources. Budget allocation to primary health care clinics in Iceland is currently reformed to make it more equitable and transparent and to serve as a single financing model for both, public and private clinics. An additional aim is to increase the number of primary care contacts and avoid the number of specialist visits. Under the reform, budget appropriation will account for age, gender, care needs based on socio-economic factors with future plans to also factor in the disease burden in setting budgets for primary care clinics.

Some countries with predominantly activity-based financing such as FFS or DRG have introduced volume thresholds to limit spending increases. In primary care, this is true for example in Germany where payment for services financed from public insurers is reduced once physicians have surpassed a quarterly defined volume threshold per practice. To limit hospital spending, some countries with activity-based financing including the Czech Republic, Israel and Germany have introduced reduced tariffs for treatment once a pre-defined level of volume is surpassed (de Lagasnerie et al., 2015). The similar principle exists in England where reduced tariffs are paid for all emergency activity beyond the 2008/09 threshold (Charlesworth et al., 2012). To reduce any incentives for hospitals to generate profits from premature discharges and higher readmission rates a number of countries including England (United Kingdom), Germany and the United States have defined conditions under which they do not pay for readmission if it occurs within a certain time span (e.g. 30 days) (Appleby et al., 2012). In Japan, where FFS is used across the health system, cost control, more efficient use resources and improvement in quality are sought through frequent updates in the fee schedule. This can include tariff reductions to disincentivise undesired activity, such as the provision of non-acute care in hospitals or activities that have seen recent volume increases. Alternatively, fees are increased to shift resources to areas with more funding needs. In the fee schedule's recent revisions, this approach was taken for obstetric, paediatric, emergency and surgical care and mental health care (OECD, 2015).

Over and above adjusting traditional modes of payment to better align them with clearly identified policy objectives, countries continue to reform payment systems more comprehensively by moving from one traditional payment mode to embarking on more significant changes in payment.

1.6. Innovations in health care provider payments

A number of OECD countries are exploring innovative ways to paying health providers by moving beyond blended or adapted approaches. In particular, three distinct payment trends presented in this publication aim to address all or some contemporary health policy objectives: improve co-ordination, improve quality and outcomes; improve efficiency (Figure 1.2). Payment innovations differ in their complexity: add-on payments which are frequently done ex-post are more limited in scope, payment innovations around bundled and population-based payments demand more full-scale reform, and are more complex in design and implementation. In the chapters that follow, this publication explores the way in which such payment reforms have been introduced in OECD countries:

Figure 1.2. Innovative payment schemes in OECD countries

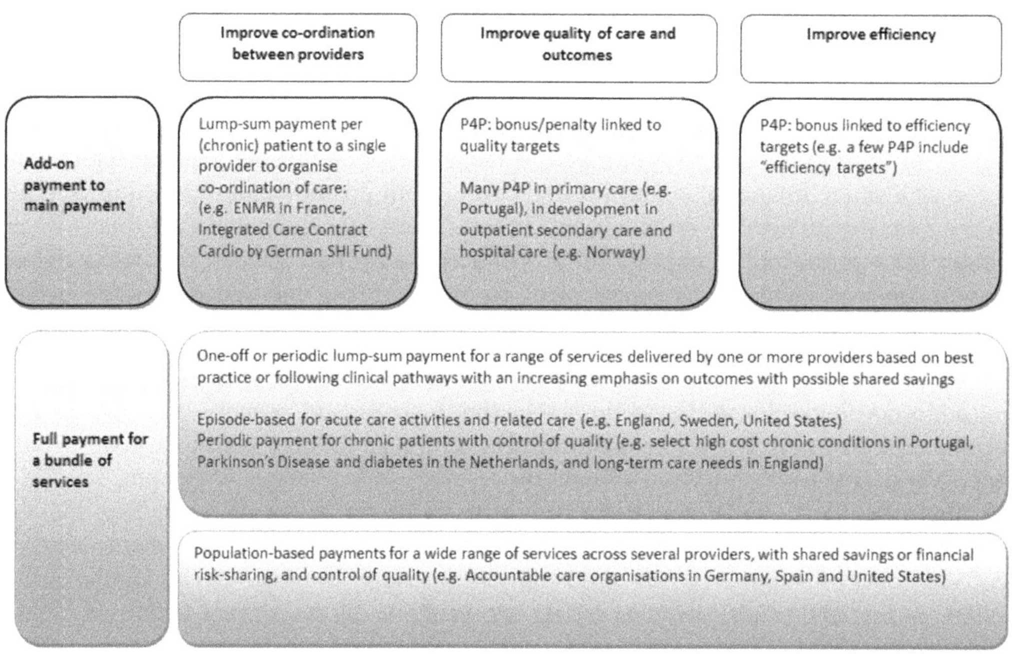

Source: Authors' compilation.

1. Add-on payments made on top of existing payment methods for co-ordination activities (as seen in France and Germany); or pay-for-performance (P4P), focussed on improving quality of care implemented in many countries (e.g. Portugal and Norway);
2. Bundled episode-based payments for specific activities of acute care based on best practice or following clinical pathways (e.g. England and Sweden); and bundled payments for the care of chronic conditions with quality requirements across delivery settings (e.g. diabetes, HIV/AIDS), as seen in the Netherlands and Portugal;
3. Population-based payment to cover a wide range of services by various providers who are encouraged to control costs and meet quality standards (e.g. United States, Germany and Spain).

1.7. Conclusion

The most commonly used traditional modes of payment, FFS, capitation, global budgets, salaries and DRGs are often poorly aligned with some of the contemporary health system priorities. Policy makers are in particular concerned that they do little to incentivise the efficient use of resources, promote the co-ordination between health providers and improve health care quality and outcomes. The strengths and weaknesses of traditional payment systems in their "pure" form led countries to respond in three ways: i) blending payment methods to counterbalance their individual shortcomings; ii) adapting traditional modes of payment in an intelligent way; iii) developing new innovative ways to pay providers.

The vast majority of countries use blended payment systems in primary care and hospital care, fewer for outpatient specialist care. In primary care, combining capitation with FFS for specific activities is frequently done. For inpatient care, the trend towards case-based financing such as DRG continues (e.g. Ireland, Greece or Israel). In many countries, hospitals receive additional financing via block grants or FFS.

Many countries have adapted their traditional payment systems to ensure they are fit for purpose. Most countries that rely on capitation payments in primary care adjust it for risk factors (e.g. age, gender, health status) to disincentivise skimping of care and cherry-picking, and the majority of them consider more than one risk dimension in their adjustment procedure. In hospitals, budget allocation is frequently done on the basis of case-mix as measured via DRGs instead of resource-based or historical budgets. Some countries with predominantly activity-based financing such as FFS or DRG have introduced volume thresholds to limit spending increases. This means that tariffs are reduced for all activity over a pre-defined level of volume. Similarly, some countries do not pay for readmission in hospitals if it occurs within a certain time span to reduce any incentives for hospitals to generate profits from premature discharges.

A number of OECD countries are exploring innovative ways to paying health providers by moving beyond blended or adapted approaches to meet health system objectives. These innovations refer to add-on payments made for co-ordination activities or to reward improvement in care quality of efficiency, bundled payments for episodes of care or for patients with chronic conditions, and population-based bundled payments where groups of providers are responsible for the delivery of all or the vast majority of health care services for a defined group of the population.

Note

1. UHI will define a standard package of services for the whole population and also introduce universal primary care, with GP care free at the point of use (Department of Health, 2012).

References

Appleby, J. et al. (2012), *Payment by Results. How Can Payment Systems Help to Deliver Better Care?*, The King's Fund, London.

Brammli-Greenberg, S. et al. (2016), "Israel Case Example – How Israel Reimburses Hospitals Based on Activity: The Procedure-related Group (PRG) Incremental Reform", submitted for the OECD Project on Payment Systems, http://www.oecd.org/health/paying-providers.htm.

Brocklehurst, P. et al. (2013), "The Effect of Different Methods of Remuneration on the Behaviour of Primary Care Dentists", *Cochrane Database of Systematic Reviews*, Vol. 11.

Busse, R. et al. (2011), *Diagnosis-Related Groups in Europe*, European Observatory on Health Systems and Policies, Open University Press, Maidenhead.

Chandra, A., D. Cutler and Z. Song (2012), "Who Ordered That? The Economics of Treatment Choices in Medical Care", in M.V. Pauly, T.G. McGuire and P.P. Barros (eds.), *Handbook of Health Economics*, Vol. 2, Elsevier Science, Amsterdam, pp. 397-432.

Charlesworth, A., A. Davies and J. Dixon (2012), *Reforming Payment for Health Care in Europe to Achieve Better Value*, Nuffield Trust, London.

de Lagasnerie, G. et al. (2015), "Tapering Payments in Hospitals: Experiences in OECD Countries", *OECD Health Working Papers*, No. 78, OECD Publishing, Paris, http://dx.doi.org/10.1787/5js4h5rlkxxr-en.

Department of Health (2013), "Money Follows the Patient – Policy Paper on Hospital Financing", Dublin, Ireland.

Department of Health (2012), "Future Health – A Strategic Framework for Reform of the Health Service 2012-2015", Dublin, Ireland.

Devlin, R.A. and S. Sarma (2008), "Do Physician Remuneration Schemes Matter? The Case of Canadian Family Physicians", *Journal of Health Economics*, Vol. 27, No. 5, pp. 1168-1181.

Dumont, E. et al. (2008), "Physicians' Multitasking and Incentives: Empirical Evidence from a Natural Experiment", *Journal of Health Economics*, Vol. 27, No. 6, pp. 1436-1450.

Economou, C. (2015), "New Prospective Hospital Reimbursement System Needs Adjustment", Update to Health in Transition profile of Greece, http://www.hspm.org/countries/greece09062014/livinghit.aspx?Section=3.6%20Payment%20mechanisms&Type=Section#2Newprospectivehospitalreimbursementsystemneedsadjustment.

European Commission (2012), "The Second Economic Adjustment Programme for Greece", *European Economy Occasional Papers No. 94*, Brussels.

Geissler, A. et al. (2011), "Introduction to DRGs in Europe: Common Objectives across Different Hospital Systems", in R. Busse, A. Geissler, W. Questin and M. Wiley (eds), *Diagnosis-related Groups in Europe – Moving Towards Transparency, Efficiency and Quality in Hospitals*, European Observatory on Health Systems and Policies Series.

Gneezy, U., S. Meier and P. Rey-Biel (2011), "When and Why Incentives (Don't) Work to Modify Behavior", *Journal of Economic Perspectives*, Vol. 25, No. 4, pp. 191-209.

Gosden, T. et al. (2003), "Paying Doctors by Salary: A Controlled Study of General Practitioner Behaviour in England", *Health Policy*, Vol. 64, No. 3, pp. 415-423.

Gosden, T. et al. (2000), "Capitation, Salary, Fee-for-service and Mixed Systems of Payment: Effects on the Behaviour of Primary Care Physicians", *Cochrane Database of Systematic Reviews 2000*, Vol. 3, Art. No. CD002215, http://dx.doi.org/10.1002/14651858.CD002215.

Health Service Executive (2014), *National Service Plan 2015*, Dublin. Ireland.

Iverson, T. (2015), "Primary Care: Effectiveness and Costs", in R.M. Scheffler (ed.), *World Scientific Handbook of Global Health Economics and Public Policy*, Vol. 3, Health System Characteristics and Performance, Imperial College Press.

Jegers, M. et al. (2002), "A Typology for Provider Payment Systems in Health Care", *Health Policy*, Vol. 60, No. 3, pp. 255-273.

Kantarevic, J. and B. Kralj (2013), "Link Between Pay for Performance Incentives and Physician Payment Mechanisms: Evidence from the Diabetes Management Incentive in Ontario", *Health Economics*, Vol. 22, No. 12, pp. 1417-1439.

Kobel, C. et al. (2011), "DRG Systems and Similar Patient Classification Systems in Europe", in R. Busse, A. Geissler, W. Questin and M. Wiley (eds), *Diagnosis-Related Groups in Europe – Moving Towards Transparency, Efficiency and Quality in Hospitals*, European Observatory on Health Systems and Policies Series.

Kwon, S. (2003), "Payment of Health Care Providers in Korea", *Health Policy and Planning*. Vol. 18, No. 1, pp. 84-92.

Kwon, S. and C. Shon (2015), "Implementation Experience with DRG-based Payment", *Asia Pacific Observatory on Health Systems and Policies Comparative Country Studies Series*, Vol. 1, No. 2, "Case-based payment systems for hospital funding in Asia – An investigation of current status and future directions".

Marshal, M. and S. Harrison (2005), "It's About More Than Money: Financial Incentives and Internal Motivation", *Quality and Safety in Health Care*, Vol. 14, pp. 4–5.

Mathauer, I. and F. Wittenbecher (2013), "Hospital Payment Systems Based on Diagnosis-related Groups: Experiences in Low- and Middle-income Countries", *Bulletin of the World Health Organization*, Vol. 91, No. 10, pp. 746-56A.

Mathauer, I. and F. Wittenbecher (2012), *DRG-based Payment Systems in Low- and Middle-income Countries: Implementation Experiences and Challenges*, World Health Organization, Geneva.

McDonald, R. et al. (2007), "Impact of Financial Incentives on Clinical Autonomy and Internal Motivation in Primary Care: Ethnographic Study", *British Medical Journal*, Vol. 334, pp. 1357-1362.

McGuire, T. (2000), "Physician Agency", in A.J. Culyer and J.P. Newhouse (eds), *Handbook of Health Economics*, Vol. 1, Elsevier Science, Amsterdam.

Melichar, L. (2009), "The Effect of Reimbursement on Medical Decision Making: Do Physicians Alter Treatment in Response to a Managed Care Incentive?", *Journal of Health Economics*, Vol. 28), pp. 902-907.

Moreno-Serra, R. and A. Wagstaff (2010), "System-wide Impacts of Hospital Payment Reforms: Evidence from Central and Eastern Europe and Central Asia", *Journal of Health Economics*, Vol. 29, pp. 585-602.

Murakami, Y. and L. Lorenzoni (2015), "Assessing the Impact of Case-based Payment", *Asia Pacific Observatory on Health Systems and Policies Comparative Country Studies Series*, Vol. 1, No. 2, "Case-based payment systems for hospital funding in Asia – An investigation of current status and future directions".

OECD (2015), *OECD Reviews of Health Care Quality: Japan: Raising Standards,* OECD Publishing, Paris, http://dx.doi.org/10.1787/9789264225817-en.

OECD (2014a), "Making Mental Health Count: The Social and Economic Costs of Neglecting Mental Health Care", OECD Health Policy Studies, OECD Publishing, Paris, http://dx.doi.org/10.1787/9789264208445-en.

OECD (2014b), "Paying Providers for Health Care. Results of the 2012 Health Systems Characteristics Survey", http://www.oecd.org/els/health-systems/paying-providers.htm.

OECD (2012), *OECD Review of Health Care Quality: Korea: Raising Standards*, OECD Publishing, Paris, http://dx.doi.org/10.1787/9789264173446-en.

Olejaz, M. et al. (2012), "Denmark: Health System Review", *Health Systems in Transition*, Vol. 14, No. 2, pp. 1-192.

Or, Z. and U. Häkinnen (2011), "DRGs and Quality: For Better or Worse?", in R. Busse, A. Geissler, W. Questin and M. Wiley (eds), *Diagnosis-related Groups in Europe – Moving Towards Transparency, Efficiency and Quality in Hospitals*, European Observatory on Health Systems and Policies Series.

Palmer, K.S. et al. (2014), "Activity-Based Funding of Hospitals and Its Impact on Mortality, Readmission, Discharge, Destination, Severity of Illness, and Volume of Care: A Systematic Review and Meta-Analysis", *PLoS ONE*, Vol. 9(10), e109975.

Paris, V., M. Devaux and L. Wei (2010), "Health Systems Institutional Characteristics: A Survey of 29 OECD Countries", *OECD Health Working Papers*, No. 50, OECD Publishing, Paris, http://dx.doi.org/10.1787/5kmfxfq9qbnr-en.

Peckham, S. and K. Gousia (2014), "GP Payment Schemes Review", Policy Research Unit in the Commissioning and the Healthcare System (PRUComm).

Polyzos, N. et al. (2013), "Reforming Reimbursement of Public Hospitals in Greece During the Economic Crisis: Implementation of a DRG System", *Health Policy*, Vol. 109, pp. 14-22.

Robinson, J.C. (2001), "Theory and Practice in the Design of Physician Payment Incentives", *Milbank Quarterly*, Vol. 79(2001), pp. 149-177.

Rudoler, D. et al. (2015), "Paying for Primary Care: A Cross-sectional Analysis of Cost and Morbidity Distributions Across Primary Care Payment Models in Ontario Canada", *Social Science and Medicine*, Vol. 124, pp. 18-28.

Schreyögg, J. et al. (2014), "Forschungsauftrag zur Mengenentwicklung nach § 17b Abs. 9 KHG", Hamburg Centre for Health Economics, https://www.gkv-spitzenverband.de/media/dokumente/krankenversicherung_1/krankenhaeuser/budgetverhandlungen/mengensteuerung/Gutachten_zur_Mengenentwicklung.pdf.

Schroeder, S. and W. Frist (2013), "Phasing out Fee-for-Service Payment", *New England Journal of Medicine*, Vol. 368, No. 21, pp. 2029-2032.

Serden, L. and M. Heurgren (2011), "Sweden: The History, Development and Current Use of DRGs", in R. Busse, A. Geissler, W. Questin and M. Wiley (eds), *Diagnosis-Related Groups in Europe – Moving Towards Transparency, Efficiency and Quality in Hospitals*, European Observatory on Health Systems and Policies Series.

Shen, J. et al. (2004), "The Effects of Payment Method on Clinical Decision-making: Physician Responses to Clinical Scenarios", *Medical Care*, Vol. 42, No. 3, pp. 297-302.

Siok Swan, T. et al. (2011), "DRGs and Cost Accounting: Which Is Driving Which?", in R. Busse, A. Geissler, W. Questin and M. Wiley (eds), *Diagnosis-Related Groups in Europe – Moving Towards Transparency, Efficiency and Quality in Hospitals*, European Observatory on Health Systems and Policies Series.

Sorbero, M. et al. (2003), "The Effect of Capitation on Switching Primary Care Physicians", *Health Services Research*, Vol. 38, pp. 191-209.

Sorensen, R.J. and J. Grytten (2003), "Service Production and Contract Choice in Primary Physician Services", *Health Policy*, Vol. 66, No. 1, pp. 73-93.

Street, A. et al. (2011), "DRG-based Hospital Payment and Efficiency: Theory, Evidence, and Challenges", in R. Busse, A. Geissler, W. Quentin and M. Wiley (eds.), *Diagnosis-Related Groups in Europe – Moving Towards Transparency, Efficiency and Quality in Hospitals*, European Observatory on Health Systems and Policies.

Chapter 2

Add-on health care provider payments

This chapter explores the implementation of additional payments for health care providers, tied to particular objectives or requirements. Specifically, it looks at how additional payments have been introduced to incentivise or facilitate co-ordination, and how they have been used to encourage improvement in performance, also known as "pay for performance" or P4P. The chapter follows a standardised analytical framework to explore policies in select OECD countries, notably the ENMR programme from France, cardiovascular disease care in Germany, the introduction of Family Health Units in Portugal, the diversification of payment methods for primary care practitioners in Ontario, Canada, and the introduction of a performance-based component to hospital budgets in Norway. Best practice and lessons for other OECD countries are highlighted, focussing on the extent to which these forms of innovative payment can be said to contribute to cost savings and quality improvement, as well as other health policy objectives.

2.1. Overview

In OECD countries, ear-marked additional payments – referred here as "add-on payments" – are used to encourage improvement in health system performance across a range of domains, including co-ordination of care, improving care quality, and strengthening management of chronic conditions. These additional payments seek to complement the existing mode of payment, but not to replace them. The payments are tied to specific expectations of the care provider, and can be made either before the actual care delivery (*ex ante*) or after (*ex post*). This chapter considers ex-post and ex-ante add-on payments used to incentivise improved co-ordination of health care activities, and ex-post performance bonuses focussing on improving quality of care, which exist in many countries. The chapter explores the use of these add-on payments, and assesses their effectiveness and utility for policy making by drawing on examples taken from countries including Australia, Canada, France, Germany, Norway, Portugal and the United Kingdom.

Instead of providing a full overview of possible add-on payments, this chapter will focus on two types of payments where there appears to be increasing policy interest in recent years: i) add-on payments used to incentivise improved co-ordination of health care activities across providers; ii) add-on payments to improve quality and efficiency where bonus payments are related to meeting pre-defined targets, also referred to as pay-for-performance (P4P) schemes.

The chapter begins by establishing the distinction between add-on payments which are applied ex-ante, and ex-post payments, which is used as one of the tools to help distinguish between different add-on payments. Then, the chapter sets out the principal case studies examined, looking first at examples of add-on payments which are used to incentivise co-ordination of care in France and in Germany. These cases are then explored following the analytical framework applied to case studies throughout this publication, assessing policy impact against the intended policy objective, across dimensions of quality, savings and unintended consequences, and considering conditions for implementation of the payment reform. Then, several examples of ex-post add-on payments are explored, P4P schemes, including examples of payment reform in Portugal, Norway, and Ontario, Canada. These payment reforms are assessed under the same framework. Finally, conclusions and lessons for OECD countries are drawn together.

Distinguishing add-on payments

Add-on payments to encourage co-ordination have been introduced in a number of OECD countries and consist of bonus payments alongside existing payment systems, such as FFS in outpatient care, and aim to give targeted incentives for particularly desirable dimensions of provider behaviour or organisation, for instance facilitating and incentivising greater collaboration across care settings and between providers. The payments can be made ex post or ex ante and are directed towards activities expected to improve co-ordination, notably establishment of a care plan, collaborative care meetings or improvements in the management of a health care structure. These types of payment can also be made to meet other health policy objectives. Additional payments for extended consultation hours to improve access to health care, for example, exist in a number of countries, but are not discussed here further.

Add-on payments, which reward quality and performance after care is delivered, are also known as P4P. P4P schemes are typically expected to improve desirable provider performance, most frequently in relation to quality or efficiency. That being said there is no internationally established or consistently applied definition of P4P to date. Indeed, P4P is often used interchangeably with terms such as "paying for results", "performance-based funding", or "results-based financing". In most definitions of P4P, performance and/or quality improvement are common themes (see Table 2.1).

Table 2.1. Definitions of pay for performance

Organisation	P4P definition
Agency for Healthcare Research and Quality (AHRQ)	Paying more for good performance on **quality metrics**
Centers for Medicare and Medicaid Services (CMS)	The use of payment methods and other incentives to encourage **quality improvement** and patient focused high value care
Rand Corporation	The general strategy of promoting **quality improvement** by rewarding providers (physicians, clinics or hospitals) who meet certain performance expectations with respect to health care **quality or efficiency**
World Bank	A range of mechanisms designed to enhance the **performance of the health system** through incentive-based payments
United States Agency for International Development (USAID)	P4P introduces incentives (generally financial) to reward attainment of **positive health results**
Center for Global Development	Transfer of money or material goods conditional on taking a **measurable action or achieving a pre-determined performance target**

Source: OECD (2010), *Value for Money in Health Spending*, OECD Publishing, Paris.

These add-ons also sit alongside existing payments systems, but unlike ex-post or ex-ante payments for co-ordination, performance payments are dependent on the provider having met certain defined objectives during service delivery. Unlike ex-ante add-on payments, which are applied prior to provision of services and/or are automatically applied to certain processes (i.e. providers understand that certain listed services will receive additional payment), add-on payments for quality are focussed on the degree of achievement of certain defined objectives by providers or practitioners, hence the "performance" dimension. The payment of the bonus, or component of the budget which is allocated based on the defined performance criteria, comes after providers have reported on the required indicators and outcomes, and are judged to have met required targets or thresholds. When providers do not meet the required targets or thresholds for the ex-post bonus, the payment is withheld.

Ex-post add-on payments are very commonly orientated towards improving quality of care and broad improvements in patient outcomes, but they can also be geared towards efficiency, such as increasing the share of prescribed generics, as well as towards improving co-ordination. Payments can be based on achievement of process indicators, for example completion of certain diagnostic tests for set patient groups, and/or on health outcomes. Usually such outcome payments are focussed on intermediate outcomes, for instance controlled blood pressure or blood glucose level, and only more rarely outcome measures such as survival rates.

Underlying and motivating P4P programmes is a desire by policy makers to assess and reward provider performance across a given domain or domains. For example, this can be an area of health care where quality of care is poor, such as chronic conditions, or where there is under-provision of services, such as preventive activities, for instance influenza vaccination for the elderly population.

P4P payments are made ex post, and have so far been applied as an add-on alongside other dominant payment methods, typically accounting for no more than 15% of total provider revenue in primary care and 12% in the outpatient sector (OECD, 2014). In the inpatient sector the share of provider revenue is much smaller, frequently around 0.1% of hospital budgets and never exceeding 4% (Milstein and Schreyögg, 2015). While P4P programmes can be expected to include at least some performance or outcome measures, most if not all P4P programmes also include simpler ex-post payments linked to service delivery (e.g. completion of certain data and recording, care plan establishment). Figure 2.1 shows a general framework for how P4P programmes are designed, including the programme measures, basis for reward, and reward. This publication focusses on provider-based financial rewards.

Figure 2.1. Framework for assessing and rewarding health care provider performance

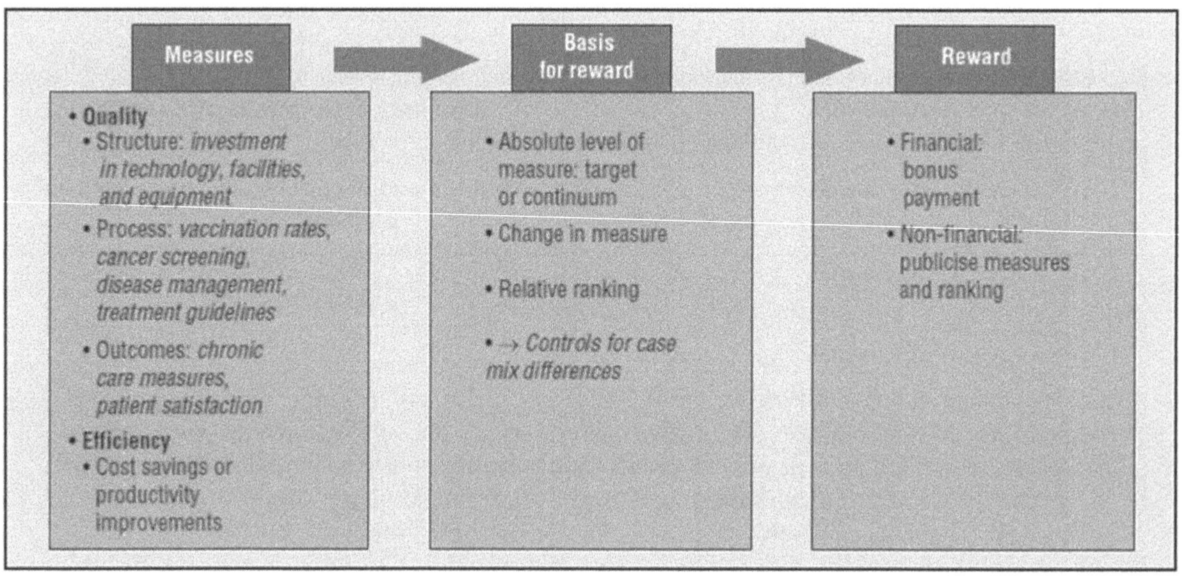

Source: OECD (2010), *Value for Money in Health Spending*, OECD Publishing, Paris.

The way in P4P programmes are set up, from the choice of indicators, setting expected targets and outcomes, to the nature of the reward (e.g. a bonus payment) will significantly affect the scope and degree of impact. The awarding of a P4P payment (reward) is based on achievement of designated targets (basis for reward). The way in which this achievement is defined varies, from absolute targets, a relative change, or a relative ranking – which are drawn from selected measures of performance, for instance quality or efficiency (structure, process or outcome). Additional aspects that influence the design of P4P programmes include whether incentives should be targeted at groups or individual health professionals, the time lag between performance and payment and the frequency of bonus payments (Cashin et al., 2014).

In many ways, add-on payments for co-ordination (and to an extent P4P) represent an evolution of FFS payments. Add-on payments for co-ordination frequently constitute an additional payment for an additional delineated activity much as FFS payments do. There are clear similarities between add-on payments for co-ordination and add-on payments for quality (P4P) and boundaries between the two can be blurred. Both have the same final objective: improving the quality of care. While add-on payments for co-ordination can be interpreted as filling gaps in the existing fee schedule, by paying desirable – but previously unrewarded services, quality-orientated P4P schemes are typically more complex and depend on the achievement of objective targets in certain domains.

This chapter follows the analytical framework applied to case studies throughout this publication, assessing policy impact against the policy objective, – across dimensions of quality and savings, as well as unintended consequences – and considering the conditions for implementation. This chapter focusses primarily on seven case studies: add-on payments to incentivise co-ordination in France (applied ex ante) and in Germany (ex post); and ex-post add-ons and examples of P4P schemes – in Australia, Canada, France, Norway, and Portugal.

2.2. Using add-on payments to encourage co-ordination

Two promising models to improve co-ordination of care

The rise in the prevalence of chronic conditions and demands of patients with complex needs has led to a need for more integrated and co-ordinated care among providers. Add-on payments – both ex ante and ex post – are being used to incentivise co-ordination of health services. Better co-ordination between care providers is seen as desirable because it can improve patient care and outcomes, and/or because better co-ordination can help to generate efficiency gains and overall cost savings. This review shows how payment is used to encourage greater co-ordination and integration of care across different levels of care in France and in Germany.

The ENMR in France

In France, add-on payments called "*Expérimentations de nouveaux modes de rémunération*" (ENMR) (Experimentation of new modes of remuneration) were introduced in 2009 (IRDES, 2013). They were made available to three different types of multi-disciplinary primary care facilities: "*maisons de santé*" (multi-professional medical home), "*pôles de santé*" (multi-professional medical facilities) and "*centres de santé*" (traditional health centre) aiming to enhance the organisation of care and providing new services to patients, and give a financial incentive for collaborative working structures. *Centres de santé* have been in operation for decades and mainly serve under-privileged urban areas. The *maisons de santé* and the *pôles de santé* were established more recently in under-served rural areas. Compared to other countries, there was a perceived lack of alternative delivery models to foster collaboration between health professionals and a need to improve working conditions for young physicians in France. The facilities included in ENMR provide primary care and sometimes secondary care as well as public health, prevention, and health education. A mix of health professionals works in these structures (e.g. doctors, midwives, nurses, pharmacists).

Add-on payments are made to the structures – and not to the professionals – which can freely decide how the fixed ENMR component is spent. All other services provided by the practice are paid in the traditional way, which is mainly FFS. Until 2014, the add-on payment was applied to three different modules: 1) co-ordinating activities, 2) provision of new services and 3) inter-professional co-operation. The activities rewarded could, for example, include the collective discussion of patient files by several health professionals. The ENMR has been modified in 2015 when the French Ministry of Health has rolled out the ENMR on a wider scale and now also foresees activities to improve access and foster the uptake of IT systems.

The ENMR component represents on average 5% of the structure's income derived from normal business and is paid by the social health insurance (CNAMTS). The regional health agencies (ARS) are responsible for selecting the structures participating in the ENMR innovation and for monitoring results. Initially, the selection criteria for structures were only vague but they have been more clearly defined since 2015. Participating facilities are now required to organise regular formalised meetings among physicians, to clearly identify one person responsible to co-ordinate care for patients, and to start digitalising patient files.

Take-up so far has varied with the majority of multi-disciplinary primary care settings signing up for the co-ordination module and 50% for new service provisions by 2014. Around 150 structures participated in the ENMR by the end of 2012, 150 more joined in 2014 when the experimentation was extended. Of the EUR 8.5 million spent on the ENMR in 2013, EUR 7.6 million were spent on co-ordinating activities (EUR 50 000 allocated per structure); spending associated with provision of new services represented EUR 950 000 across all structures. In 2015, the French Ministry of Health generalised the ENMR and widened its scope to cover new multi-disciplinary settings. Compared to the first wave of ENMR experimentation there are some modifications with regards to payment, consisting now of fixed and variable bonus payments for required and optional activities. The ministry estimates that associated spending will reach EUR 50 million by 2017, covering 1 000 structures with 10 000 health professionals co-ordinating care for 4 million patients (Ministère des Affaires Sociales, 2015).

Integrated care contracts in Germany

Integration of care across different health sectors was introduced in German social law in the year 2000. Previously, cross-sectoral co-operation, for example, between primary care physicians and hospitals, was not very well developed. In this context, integration of care refers to programmes set up by individual health insurers mainly to improve health care quality for their insured through improved co-operation among different health providers. The legislative changes serve as the legal basis for Statutory Health Insurance Funds to *selectively* contract health providers for the provision of health services and the integrated care programmes. The German health system is typically characterised by *collective* contracting between all Statutory Health Insurers and health provider associations. In 2011, around 6 300 different contracts for integrated care programmes existed. The high number can be explained by the high number of Statutory Health Insurance Funds (118 in 2016) and the fact that integrated care contracts are predominantly signed at a regional level. One example of an integrated care contract is the "Cardio-Integral" programme launched by the Statutory Health Insurance Fund "AOK Plus" in 2005 (Milstein and Blankart, 2016). The main objectives of the programme is a closer co-operation between GPs and specialists across ambulatory and inpatient care, the linkage to a Disease Management Program (DMP), a reduction in waiting times and the realisation of efficiency gains by better care co-ordination. The closer co-operation should also lead to better care quality by improved diagnostic, therapy and follow-up care.

All patients with cardiovascular diseases living in Saxony and insured by AOK Plus are eligible to participate in the programme. Contracting partners are a regional association of GPs, the Heart Centre of the University Hospital Dresden and an outpatient clinic of the University Hospital Dresden. Outpatient specialists can also join the contract. All health providers are eligible to receive add-on payments for co-ordinating additional services associated with the programme such as preparing patients for invasive surgery (Milstein and Blankart, 2016). GPs and specialists have to meet some minimal requirements to participate in this programme, for example, they need access to a 24-hour, blood-pressure-measuring instrument and have to be willing to participate in the programme evaluation.

Patients are treated according to defined care pathways which differ depending on the cardiovascular condition. Both GPs and outpatient specialists have a co-ordination role. Non-invasive specialists decide about the potential participation of patients in the programme, and co-ordinate care between GPs and specialist clinics and hospitals in case invasive treatment is required. Together with invasive specialists, they establish therapeutic plans and define treatment targets and refer patients back to GPs. GPs supervise patient's adherence to protocol and monitor targets. Extensive exchange of data between health providers is required in the programme.

In 2010, there were about 50 000 patients enrolled in the programme, about 1 200 GPs and 91 specialists participating with a total budget of EUR 2.4 million.

Improvements in quality and lower costs

In both France and Germany, add-on payments are associated with an improvement in the quality of care provided and reductions in health spending, although it is difficult to establish clear causality. In France, the multi-disciplinary structures achieve better results for nearly all care indicators (e.g. diabetes care processes, prevention and efficient prescription) than traditional practices but they were already performing better before the introduction of the ENMR (IRDES, 2014a). However, for some indicators, the difference in performance between multi-disciplinary structures and traditional practices has grown with the introduction of the payment innovation. The most significant improvement for multi-disciplinary structures relates to better control for HbA1c levels. Costs in multidisciplinary structures were between 0.5% and 2.3% lower for spending on specialists, nurses, physiotherapy and pharmaceuticals than in traditional practices. But again, the cost differences pre-date the introduction of the payment scheme. Multi-disciplinary settings are more efficient than traditional practices, particularly for the more integrated *maisons de santé*, where doctors see significantly more patients and perform more services. Multi-disciplinary practice is motivated by improved working conditions for health professionals and the add-on payments led to more effective organisation of care through greater collaboration and co-ordination between health professionals (IRDES, 2014a).

Similarly, positive results were found with the Cardio-Integral programme in Germany for patients with cardiovascular disease. There has been a reduction in repeat examination and better patient-centered collaboration between doctors. About 89% of patients acknowledge better co-operation between the GP and cardiologist and 65% of patients report an improvement in their health status after enrollment. GPs and specialists highlight the good quality and completeness of patient data. Hence, the vast majority of providers and patients are satisfied with the programme (Werblow and Karmann, 2012). However, patients still perceive relatively long waiting times for specialist treatment to be an issue although doctors report that Cardio-Integral patients have quicker access to specialists[1]. Werblow and Karmann (2012) find higher initial costs for patients enrolled in the programme compared to a control group. Nevertheless, the programme was able to generate savings after four and a half years. Part of the higher initial costs is due to an additional outpatient examination which is part of the enrollment procedure and changes in medication. The subsequent estimated annual savings were about EUR 96 per enrolled patient due to improved drug therapy and better post-acute treatment which helped to bring down inpatient costs for invasive interventions and heart failure. However, it is difficult to separate out the contribution of the add-on payment provided under the "Cardio-Integral" contract as it overlaps with a DMP for cardiovascular diseases (Milstein and Blankart, 2016). The DMP also foresees additional financial incentives for providers (mainly GPs) to deliver evidence-based care.

Payment experimentation accompanied by additional health reforms

In France and Germany, the introduction of add-on payments was part of broader health reforms which contributed to the ease of their implementation. In France, the implementation of the ENMR complemented other health policy reforms such as the introduction of the P4P scheme CAPI/ROSP,[2] which was introduced around the same time. In Germany, the Cardio-Integral contract is an application of a change in the federal social code allowing selective contracting between individual health insurance funds and individual or groups of health providers for care delivery models across sectors. Insurers and providers can freely negotiate the nature of integrated services and the way they are paid. In both countries, voluntary participation among providers and patients in the new model appears to be another factor contributing to success. Providers have responded favourably to the innovation in both settings. Patients are free to decide whether they want to participate in the Cardio-Integral in Germany. In France, patients automatically benefit from better co-ordination if they choose to consult one of the structures where the ENMR is implemented.

Payments can target provider structures or physicians

In France, until 2014 nearly all multi-disciplinary settings signed up for the co-ordination module of the ENMR payment, and 50% signed up for the new service provisions module. The third module became operational in 2014. The ENMR payment for each structure was calculated separately for each module. Module one (co-ordinating activities) took into account the number of full-time equivalent staff and the number of patients indicating a "médecin traitant"[3] (primary physician). For ENMR-module 2 (provision of new services), the number of patients was considered, and for ENMR-module 3 (inter-professional co-operation), the number of nurses (IRDES, 2013). In most cases, these resources were used to pay the time dedicated for co-ordinating services by health professionals, to purchase IT equipment or to strengthen the management of the sites (IRDES, 2014b). With the extension of the ENMR in 2014 and the generalisation of the innovation in 2015, the mode of payment of the ENMR has been modified. For the co-ordination module, required and optional activities have been defined and for both, a fixed and variable bonus payment has been developed. The payment continues to take into account the number of patients but also reflects achievement in improving co-ordination, access of care and the uptake of IT. This refers, for example, to the development of treatment protocols within the structure or the extension of consultation hours. The structure receives 60% of the expected payment as an advance in the spring of the current year with the remaining part being withheld to take into account any possible adjustments in payments.

At its outset, the ENMR was planned to reward performance and not structural features. Initially, performance per group practice should have been measured on the basis of a number of indicators covering the dimensions quality of care, co-ordination and efficient prescription. However, the idea to link ENMR payments to performance was dropped for practical reasons, principally measurement and reporting problems.

In the German Cardio-Integral, programme-specific tariffs and activities are negotiated between insurers and participating providers. Add-on payments for the Cardio-Integral programme are available to GPs for regular check-ups, monitoring tasks, and preparing patients for an invasive intervention (EUR 20-40). Specialists receive add-on payments for patient enrollment and for co-ordinating with GPs and invasive specialists (EUR 20-80). Depending on the service bonus payments can be made quarterly, bi-annually or annually.

In both countries, add-on payments represent additional sources of revenue for providers and are not a mere reallocation of existing funds. This appears to be one factor in the overall support of providers to this innovation, although the available payments account for 5% or less of total provider income. In the case of Cardio-Integral in Germany, the financial incentive has been identified as the main motivation for specialists to join the programme (Werblow and Karmann, 2012). Both payment innovations are associated with additional administrative work for health providers, but the additional administration burden of these innovations for participating health care providers is relatively small compared to more advanced payment reforms such as P4P, bundled or population-based payments.

Add-on payment for co-ordination are easy to implement but limited in scope

Overall, add-on payments for co-ordination are relatively easy to implement and generally require fewer IT investments and data exchanges compared to the more sophisticated payment innovations where payments rely on the measurement of patient metrics. Incremental changes within the general payment structure are likely to face less provider resistance than more thorough payment reforms where financial consequences for providers are more difficult to anticipate. In France and Germany, providers supported the introduction of add-on payments. The administrative burden of these innovations can be expected to be comparably small. The scope of these incentives is limited as they focus on the improvement of co-operation of health professionals within and across provider settings. This approach seems to support the provision of seamless care and enhance care quality, but unlike in many P4P schemes, which usually include a broad suite of more output-oriented indicators, the focus of the add-ons for co-ordination remains on incentivising specific behaviours at specific points of the care pathway.

Similar incentives exist also in other countries (The Commonwealth Fund, 2015). To promote care integration and care provision from single practices to group practices consisting of multi-disciplinary teams, some Italian regions pay GPs an add-on to the regular capitated amounts. They are expected to collaborate with specialists, nurses and social workers. In Australia, there are additional incentive payments targeted at practice nurses for co-ordinating activities.

2.3. Add-on payments to reward quality and outcomes

Add-on payments which reward quality and performance, known as P4P, also sit alongside existing payments systems. Unlike add-on payments for co-ordination, which can be applied ex ante to provision of services and/or are automatically applied to certain processes, P4P payments are applied ex post. They are allocated after providers have reported on the required indicators and outcomes, and are deemed to have met the required targets or thresholds. They are focussed on the degree of achievement of specific defined objectives by providers or practitioners. P4P has emerged as one potential lever to address some of the shortcomings of traditional payments of FFS, capitation, and salary. P4P is typically an add-on payment which promotes evidence-based and preventive services that are linked to specific "targets".

Add-on P4P payments are widespread across OECD countries, and beyond. In 2012, nearly two-thirds of OECD countries reported having at least one P4P scheme in place (OECD, 2014). The popularity of P4P schemes also appears to be increasing; the number of countries reporting such schemes also rose between 2008 and 2012. Based on responses for the OECD Health Systems Characteristics Surveys (2008 and 2012), the largest number of P4P programmes are found in primary care, but P4P are also spreading to specialists and acute hospitals. Between the 2008 and 2012 Health Systems Characteristics Surveys, three P4P schemes were introduced in primary care (Korea, Mexico, Netherlands), three to specialist care (France, Korea, Netherlands), and seven to acute care (Australia, France, Korea, New Zealand, Portugal, Spain, Sweden) (OECD Health Systems Characteristics Survey, 2012; OECD, 2014; Paris et al., 2010). Beyond this, performance-based payment is also being introduced in more diverse care settings, for example long-term care in the United States (CMS, 2015) and public health and prevention outside of GP practices such as for delivery of vaccination services or smoking cessation in pharmacies in the United Kingdom (see Box 2.1). Pharmacy services and their payment arrangements are also evolving in Australia. The Pharmacy Trial Programme will expand the role of community pharmacies in the delivery of primary health care services to collaborate with GPs and other practitioners to improve clinical outcomes of patients (Department of Health, 2016b). The design of the trial programmes and associated payment arrangement will be primarily developed by the organisations putting forward the trial idea, as well as expert advisory groups.

Box 2.1. Performance-based payment incentives for smoking cessation programmes in England

England has been developing ways to apply performance incentives to broader parts of the health service, including developing "payment-by-results" contracts for smoking cessation programmes in a series of pilots from 2010. The objective of this approach was to increase the uptake of high-quality smoking cessation services, and to encourage stop-smoking services to increase their supply of services. Contracts were made with NHS providers, third sector charity and private providers (e.g. pharmacies), for services including assessment, counselling, and follow-up.

The design of the payment incentive varies slightly between schemes and contracts, but the overriding principle is that providers receive an initial payment for the service, followed by further payment provided that the client has not resumed smoking within a set follow-up period.

In one scheme, a bonus payment of GBP 30.50 was made for each new client accessing the service who has their smoking status recorded four weeks after their "quit date" (regardless of whether the person has quit smoking or not), and a further GBP 30 bonus for every person who has quit after four weeks, verified with a carbon monoxide (CO) monitor. An additional bonus of GBP 50 is made for every person who is still not smoking after 12 weeks. A different scheme worked on a very similar basis, with a slightly different bonus structure, and also offered an enhanced tariff for a target population (in this case, identified hard to reach groups including black and minority ethnicities, and lower socioeconomic groups).

A full evaluation has not yet been published, but preliminary results suggest some positive results, both in terms of quit rate and rate at which CO and quit status is recorded. A cluster controlled study found positive results also, suggesting that payment scheme has helped improve the effectiveness and supply of NHS stop smoking services, having incentivised specific clinical outcomes and contributed towards attracting new service providers.

Source: McLeod et al. (2015), Department of Health (2016a).

In OECD countries, P4P schemes are most common in primary care (14 countries) followed by inpatient care (11 countries) and then outpatient specialist care (seven countries) (see Tables 2.2 and 2.3). In primary care, bonuses are paid most frequently for the achievement of targets relating to preventive care and the management of chronic diseases, less often for the uptake of IT initiatives, patient satisfaction or efficient care provision (e.g. share of generic medicines prescribed). In the majority of countries, bonus payments are made to the individuals based on the achievement of absolute targets. In hospitals, P4P targets relate most commonly to patient experience, clinical outcomes and the use of appropriate processes. In most OECD countries, hospital performance is measured either as absolute targets or observed changes over time.

Table 2.2. Payment for performance activities in primary care and outpatient specialist care

Participation of health providers	Country	P4P target typically relates to						Bonus payment is made to		Performance measurement		
		Preventive care	Management chronic diseases	Uptake of IT services	Patient satisfaction	Efficiency	Other	Individual	Organisation	Absolute	Change over time	Relative ranking
		Primary care										
Mandatory participation	Chile	●	●	○	●	●	●	●	○	●	○	○
	Korea	○	●	○	○	●	○	●	○	○	●	●
	Spain	●	●	○	○	●	○	●	○	●	●	○
	Sweden	●	●	●	●	●	○	○	●	●	●	●
	Turkey	●	○	○	○	●	●	●	○	●	○	○
Voluntary participation with conditions	Australia	●	●	●	○	○	●	●	●	●	○	○
	France	●	●	●	○	●	○	●	○	○	●	○
	Mexico	●	●	○	●	●	●	●	○	○	○	●
	New Zealand	●	●	○	○	○	○	○	●	●	●	○
	Portugal	●	●	○	●	●	○	●	○	●	○	○
	United States	●	●	●	●	●	○	●	●	●	●	●
Voluntary open participation	Czech Republic	●	○	○	○	○	●	●	○	○	○	●
	Hungary	●	●	○	○	●	○	○	●	●	○	○
	United Kingdom	●	●	○	●	●	○	○	●	●	○	○
		Outpatient specialist care										
Mandatory participation	Chile	●	●	○	○	○	●	●	○	●	○	○
	Korea	○	●	○	○	○	○	●	○	○	●	●
	Spain	○	●	●	●	●	○	●	○	●	●	○
Voluntary participation with conditions	France	○	○	●	○	○	●	●	○	○	●	○
	United States	●	●	●	●	●	○	●	●	●	●	●

Note: Estonia and the Netherlands also use P4P in primary care but did not provide additional information. The Netherlands and the United Kingdom also use P4P for outpatient specialist care but did not provide additional information.

Source: Questions 37 and 38 from the OECD Health Systems Characteristics Survey 2012, and OECD Secretariat's estimates.

Table 2.3. Payment for performance activities in inpatient care

Participation of health providers	Country	P4P target typically relate to					Performance measurement		
		Clinical outcomes of care	Use of appropriate processes	Patient satisfaction	Patient experience	Other	Absolute measurement	Change over time	Relative ranking
Mandatory participation	Australia	○	○	○	●	○	○	●	○
	France	○	○	○	○	●	○	○	○
	Korea	●	●	○	○	○	●	●	●
	Spain	●	●	○	●	○	●	●	○
	Sweden	●	●	○	●	○	●	●	●
	Portugal	●	●	●	●	○	●	○	○
	Turkey	○	●	○	●	○	●	○	○
Voluntary open participation	Luxembourg	○	○	○	○	●	●	○	○
	United Kingdom	●	●	●	●	○	●	●	○
Mandatory and voluntary	United States	●	●	●	●	○	●	●	●

Note: Netherlands has a hospital P4P programme, but no additional information was provided. The category "other" refers to hospital management in Luxembourg and the efficient use of medication in France. Patient satisfaction refers to subjective appreciation on the quality of care and accommodation. Patient experience refers to waiting times, information given by medical staff, etc.

Source: Questions 39 from the OECD Health Systems Characteristics Survey 2012 and OECD Secretariat's estimates.

This chapter does not give a full account of P4P programmes across OECD countries, as a comprehensive review can be found in the recent joint OECD publication with the European Observatory and the French Health Insurance Fund (CNAMTS) (see Cashin et al., 2014). Instead, this chapter focusses on new features of more recent P4P schemes, and reflects on the relationship between P4P schemes and other payments systems, both innovative and traditional.

Different approaches to paying for improvements in the care of diabetic patients are also considered, looking at P4P schemes in Australia, Germany and France. This special focus on diabetes is introduced to draw out first, how highly prevalent chronic diseases are an important focus of P4P add-ons, secondly to demonstrate how there are quite significant differences between P4P programmes even when applied to the same condition and expected treatment approach, and thirdly to present in more detail the construction of incentives targeted at one specific area of health care performance.

Reforming GP practice in Ontario, Canada and diversifying payment methods

In Ontario, Canada, P4P was introduced to primary care practitioners as part of a wider diversification of payment mechanisms. In the late 1990s, Ontario inaugurated "Primary Care Reform" characterised by the sequential introduction of a "menu" of payment models replacing traditional FFS payment for family physicians. This reform was brought about by, in part, concerns regarding a shortage of family physicians and about access to physicians during evenings and weekends. Improving health care quality, for example increasing the payment system's support for preventative health care and chronic disease management, was also an important goal. The FFS payment system was seen as contributing towards an excessive focus on volume-based acute care, and to lack incentives encouraging both physician and inter-professional teams (Kantarevic and Kralj, 2015).

Over time, the reform introduced a menu of blended primary care payment models, employing various combinations of FFS, capitation, P4P in the form of incentives and bonuses, and/or salary. Physicians were given a choice of payment model. These newly introduced models required or encouraged patient enrollment (sometimes called rostering) with GPs. For most models, physicians practiced in groups of at least three and shared records but need not be co-located. Higher level objectives of the reform included improved access, quality and continuity of care (Sweetman and Buckley, 2014). The take-up of these new contracts has been significant: while in 1998, almost 100% of primary care physicians were paid by traditional FFS; this proportion had dropped to approximately 37% by 2009/10, and further still to approximately 30% by 2013.

The introduction of new physician payment models in Ontario was integrated with many other primary care initiatives, such as primary care models involving allied health professionals (e.g., the "Family Health Team" interdisciplinary model and Nurse Practitioner-led clinics), educational campaigns on when it is appropriate to go to an Emergency Department, when and where to seek urgent (but not emergency) care, and initiatives aimed at helping patients to find a family doctor if they did not have one (Health Care Connect programme) (Sweetman and Buckley, 2016).

The new voluntary payment schemes introduced following the Primary Care Reform target all primary care physicians practicing family medicine/primary health care, and family physicians can join at any time (with some administrative delays). The most common models, and their basic payment composition, are listed below. For instance, Family Health Organizations (blended capitation, FFS and P4P) and Family Health Groups (blended FFS and P4P) account for about 55% of primary care physicians (Table 2.4).

Table 2.4. Payment models for primary care physicians in Ontario, Canada, 2009/10

Payment model in Ontario	Percentage of primary care physicians participating	Primary method of remuneration
Traditional Fee-for-service - FFS	37%	~85% FFS (rest: salary/capitation/benefits and premiums/fees)
Family Health Organization - FHO	29%	~70% salary/capitation/benefits (rest: FFS, premiums/fees, bonus and flowthrough)
Family Health Group - FHG	26%	~80% FFS (rest: salary/capitation/benefits, premiums/fees and bonus)
Comprehensive Care Model - CCM	3%	~75% FFS (rest: salary/capitation/benefits, premiums/fees and bonus)
Family Health Network - FHN	3%	~65% salary/capitation/benefits (rest: FFS, premiums/fees, bonus and flowthrough)
Rural and Northern Physician Group Agreement - RNPGA	1%	~75% salary/capitation/benefits (rest: FFS, premiums/fees, bonus)

Note: "Flow through" indicates funds that pass through the practice to others who receive final payment.

Source: Henry, D. et al. (2012), "Payments to Ontario Physicians from Ministry of Health and Long-Term Care Sources 1992/93 to 2009/10 – ICES Investigative Report", ICES, Toronto, http://www.ices.on.ca/~/media/Files/Atlases-Reports/2012/Payments-to-Ontario-physicians-from-MOHLTC-sources/Full%20report.ashx.

All primary care incentives/bonuses in Ontario are process-based, and none are outcome-based. Additionally, some incentives are paid periodically (e.g., once a year) while others are paid every time a specific service is provided. Eligibility for some incentives is patient-based (i.e., the physician receives a payment for having provided a specific service to an individual patient), while for other incentives, eligibility is based on performance across all registered patients practice-wide (i.e., the physician receives a payment for having reached a pre-defined target level based on a number of services, a number of patients or a percentage of eligible patients who received the service). The various models differ in their eligibility for incentives.

Across the different models, the incentives include the following:

- Bonus for smoking cessation counselling;
- Bonuses for toddler immunisations, Pap smears, mammograms, influenza immunisations for seniors, and fecal occult blood test (FOBT). Payments are made yearly, and their actual amount depends on the level reached for the performance measure. For instance, payment thresholds are based on the percentage of the eligible population who received the service: e.g., variable payments dependent on the total percentage of rostered seniors who have received flu immunisation, with a higher percentage of immunisations leading to a higher payment;
- Chronic disease management: payment of CAD 60 per year for managing a patient's diabetes by monitoring levels using a tracking sheet (above and beyond payment for individual services);
- Annual payment for enrolling a fixed number of patients with serious mental illnesses, which can be cumulative if patients with a serious mental illness are already enrolled;

- Special fixed payments for providing services in hospitals and, long-term care homes. Also, special payment for providing particular services such as prenatal care, home visits, labour and deliveries, palliative care, and a minimum number of services from a list of office-based minor surgical procedures. For instance, payment of graduated thresholds between CAD 1 500 and CAD 8 000 for home visits.

It is largely unknown which of these combinations of the payment scheme is delivering the best outcomes as only a few evaluations have been completed at this point. Moreover, it is not clear that any single model dominates in all contexts. A 2013 evaluation by Li et al. suggested that P4P incentives led to only a modest improvement in performance with respect to Pap smears, mammograms, senior flu shots, and colorectal cancer screenings, and no improvement with respect to toddler immunisations. In contrast, Kantarevic and Kralj (2013), and Kiran et al. (2014), find evidence of improved primary care diabetes management. Furthermore the Ontario Government is considering other potential changes to primary care reform including payment reform but the GPs are resisting further changes. It remains to be seen whether further reform will be implemented (Marchildon and Hutchison, 2016).

P4P in Portugal led to building new primary care models of delivery

In Portugal, satisfaction with primary care was low among stakeholders, and there was particular policy interest in improving productivity and quality at the system level, including through the strengthening of primary care. The traditional working style in primary care is of GPs operating relatively independently, even when GPs are co-located in a single physical site (the traditional Primary Health Care Centres). Moving away from solo practices, a new model of primary care centre was created in 2006 – a Family Health Unit (FHU). FHUs are made up of three to eight GPs, the same number of primary care nurses, and a variable number of administrative staff, who were invited to volunteer to form self-selecting groups who deliver primary care together to patients registered with the FHU. FHUs were intended to encourage more multidisciplinary team working, and collaboration between doctors, nurses and administrative staff (Lourenço, 2016).

The average FHU has around 12 000 patients, seven doctors and 20 professionals in total (OECD, 2015). These teams have functional and technical autonomy and a payment system sensitive to performance that is designed to reward productivity, accessibility and quality, with core indicators used to measure performance and tied to the payment system.

Started as a pilot in 2005, the number of FHUs has been increasing steadily since their introduction. FHUs now cover more than 50% of the population, and all patients are eligible to register with a FHU. The FHUs cover primary care services, including services such as nursing services, home visits, etc. Provider participation is voluntary with set criteria on the composition and number of health professionals in each unit. The government is the payer via regional primary care organisations (ACES).

There are two operational models of FHU (Models A and B), with slightly distinct organisational structures and payment methods. Notably, only Model B FHUs have an individual P4P component in their payment method. Model A and Model B FHUs can also access some add-on payments for additional services and a structural P4P component for the group of providers used for quality improvement (e.g. training, equipment, infrastructure, vehicles).

All FHUs start as Model A FHUs, and must prove that they are meeting specific quality, clinical, and functional targets before they are allowed to apply to transition to

Model B. In addition to Models A and B FHUs, a third model – Model C – was developed principally as an avenue for private sector providers (for profit as well as not-for-profit) to participate in the FHU scheme. At the time of writing, no Model C units had been created.

- Model A, 212 FHUs in 2014 (OECD, 2015): All of the Model A FHU's personnel payment is governed by the public administration's legislation for the correspondent sector and profession (e.g. legislation affecting GP salary, primary care nurse salary). FHUs can also negotiate with the contracting agency (typically the ACES/Region) to agree a certain set of objectives or deliverables, the achievement of which leads to additional financing for the FHU. These objectives typically include additional services that the unit will provide, or facilities' improvements (e.g. adding disabled access facilities), and do not include individual reward for performance on indicators.

- Model B, 181 FHUs in 2014 (OECD, 2015): FHUs can progress from Model A to Model B, with the approval of the relevant ACES/Region. The payment process for Model B FHUs has two components: a fixed component and a variable one. The fixed component corresponds to the legislated payment. The variable component, which is one of the main distinctions between Models A and B, combines all supplementary payments that the FHU can receive based on the health professional's performance, and the unit's results, across a selection of indicators.

Staff working in the traditional primary care clinics (Primary Health Care Centres) in Portugal, which still cover close to 50% of the population, are salaried. In Model A, payment remains mostly by salary, but a financial incentive component is included for the whole FHU, which is usually an add-on payment/grant for accomplishing 22 key performance indicators revised every three years from a comprehensive set of more than 100 quality and efficiency indicators (Administração Central do Sistema de Saúde, 2015). In addition to Model A features, FHU Model B staff payment is composed of a smaller fixed salary fraction plus a series of supplements: a capitation-based payment (up to a defined ceiling); a complement for the provision of specific negotiated and contracted services; a FFS component for house calls; and a P4P (da Silva Fialho et al., 2008). In Model B FHUs, the performance-based payment component can reach up to 30% of total physician payment and up to 10% for nurses and is based on the achievement of individual and practice targets.

P4P in Norway aims to improve quality and outcomes in the hospital sector

Norway has introduced a P4P component to payment in Norway's four hospital regions called Quality Based Financing (QBF) (Beck Olsen and Brandborg, 2016). The introduction of QBF came as part of a broader push towards developing a more patient-centered health care service, with increased emphasis on systematic quality improvement, patient safety and reduction in adverse events. Along with QBF, the following elements (amongst others) were proposed: more active patient and user role; greater transparency around quality and patient safety; more systematic testing of new treatment methods; and the promotion of better quality through knowledge and innovation. The Directorate of Health, hospital regions, Norwegian Medical Association, Norwegian Nurses Organisation and the Norwegian Federation of Organisations of Disabled People were key stakeholders involved in designing the P4P policy.

Norway is divided into four health regions, which fund hospitals locally. These four hospital regions are commissioning and governing bodies which include all public secondary care providers and some private hospitals. Each year, funding is distributed to the four health regions by central Norwegian authorities under the Regional Health

Authority (RHA) grant. Before 2014, hospitals were financed through a mix of block grants (capitation-based – adjusted for age, several health indicators, and social indicators, and cost-adjusted for the region), and activity-based financing (DRGs) which represented close to 25% of the global budget. The new payment scheme based on quality, supplements these existing financing systems. The QBF component represents 0.5% (roughly NOK 500 million) of total funding.

The QBF component is a reflection of individual hospital's performance on the selected indicators, but the income is initially distributed at the health region level. The QBF scheme uses a point system where each RHA is attributed points based on how well hospitals perform on a set of 33 quality indicators, drawn from the National Quality Indicator System (NQIS) which was established in 2012, and a set of performance criteria. Using the NQIS, which was already being used in hospitals, meant avoiding introducing additional bureaucracy as part of the scheme. After a review, some NQIS indicators were excluded due to uncertainty in reporting quality or because the performance on the indicators was considered to be affected by factors beyond the control of the secondary care provider.

The scheme is based on outcome, process and patient satisfaction indicators. The indicators measuring patient satisfaction come from the National Patient Satisfaction Survey which is developed by and conducted by the Norwegian Knowledge Centre. Each category of indicator is weighted to reflect their relative importance (50 000 points for outcome indicators; 20 000 points for process indicators; 30 000 points for patient satisfaction). Four different criteria are used to measure and reward performance: reporting quality, minimum performance level, best performance and best relative improvement. A mix of relative performance and absolute targets are used. Absolute targets have been set in a number of areas such as cancer survival, thrombolysis and obstetrics. For instance, for the indicator "Perineal tear 3rd and 4th degree", the target was 2.3% of all vaginal births in 2015. A region reporting a higher rate will not earn points for this indicator.

Due to a time lag in the reporting and quality control of the indicators, the RHAs receive the payment two years after the activities on which the performance measurements are based. This means for example that activities that were carried out in 2012 are rewarded financially through the P4P scheme in 2014. The level of payment in the P4P scheme is set deliberately low at the start of the programme to avoid gaming and crowding out intrinsic motivation.

Since the scheme is a pilot, the government requested that an evaluation be carried out. The results of the evaluation will aid the government in determining whether the scheme will be implemented on a more permanent basis after 2016. If it is to be continued, the results from the evaluation will contribute to an adjustment of the scheme.

Focus on diabetes: Different approaches are taken in designing P4P to address quality of care for diabetes patients

Even if policy objectives are similar and the targeted disease is the same, the design of P4P programmes differs between countries and between care settings. This "special focus" on diabetes is introduced to draw out first, how highly prevalent chronic diseases are an important focus of P4P add-ons, and second, to demonstrate how there are quite significant differences between P4P programmes even when applied to the same condition and expected treatment approach, and third to present in more detail the construction of incentives targeted at one specific area of health care performance. Australia, France and Germany have introduced modifications to their predominantly FFS payment system in the last decade, particularly to facilitate the implementation of care programmes conceived around patients with diabetes. All three countries have opted to use add-on payments to reward performance of health professionals – unlike the Netherlands which moved toward bundled payments for this condition (see Chapter 3 of this publication) – to improve quality of diabetes care.

In the case of Australia and France, indicators related to diabetic care for patients with type 2 diabetes were introduced as part of broader P4P scheme; in Germany, DMPs targeted at types 1 and 2 diabetes were developed. These schemes all seek to push providers towards delivering high-quality diabetic care. This is done either by identifying and directly rewarding the activities that should be performed or by specifying and rewarding the desired outcomes. The activities set out in the programmes and their outcomes were defined by national authorities and drawn from national clinical guidelines for the treatment of diabetes.

In all three countries, incentive payments for the treatment of type 2 diabetes patients are typically directed at GPs, although specialists can be involved with some standard check-ups (e.g. ophthalmologists for eye examination), and in cases of complications (e.g. cardiologists or nephrologists). The design of the P4P framework in Australia, France and Germany, however, differs.

In Australia, bonus payments for diabetic care are one incentive area of the Practice Incentive Program (PIP). The PIP was implemented in 1998, initially focusing on 13 incentive areas which can be divided into three streams: quality of care, capacity and rural support. GPs need to fulfil certain requirements to participate in the PIP.

Under the PIP, three types of additional payments can be received by GPs for diabetic care:

- A sign-on bonus (a one-off payment for practices which sign up for the PIP Diabetes initiative);
- A so-called "Outcome" payment (an annual bonus payment if 50% of all patients with diabetes registered at the practice complete a cycle of care);
- Service Incentive Payment (an annual bonus payment for each completed cycle of care).

Whereas the sign-on payment and the outcome payment are made at the practice level, the service incentive payment (SIP) is made to the individual GP. In financial terms, the SIP is the most important bonus. It can be claimed by GPs for each cycle of care completed for patients with diagnosed diabetes. A cycle needs to be completed over a period of at least 11 months and up to 13 months. The SIP defines minimum requirements for 13 activities that need to be met under a cycle of care, for example measuring blood pressure at least twice over the cycle. The minimum required services can be provided by the GP himself or delegated to a practice nurse or other health professionals. The bonus is paid in addition to the consultation fee that the GP charges (Wong et al., 2016; Department of Human Services, 2013).

For insulin-dependent patients and patients with abnormal review findings, complications, and/or co-morbidities, additional levels of care are required. In general, the minimum requirements are based on the guidelines on diabetes management in general practice issued by the Royal Australian College of General Practitioners (RACGP) and Diabetes Australia.

In France, a number of different programmes have been established to improve diabetic care outcomes. Diabetes (types 1 and 2) is one of 30 listed long-term conditions (ALD). The physicians selected as the "médecin traitant" receives an additional annual payment for patients diagnosed with an ALD. This payment covers the care co-ordination required to implement specific care protocols. The care protocol of a patient lists all medical and paramedical services required for a comprehensive treatment, and automatically identifies the services for which patients are exempt from co-payment. In nearly all cases, this co-ordinating role is fulfilled by GPs.

A P4P scheme, initially introduced in 2009 as the *Contrat d'Amélioration des Pratiques Individuelles* (CAPI, Contract to improve individual practices), and now known as the *Rémunération sur Objectifs de Santé Publique* (ROSP, Remuneration of public health objectives) incentivises improvements in quality of care and more efficient prescribing. Currently, the ROSP includes 29 indicators from four different areas: organisation of practice, chronic conditions, prevention and efficiency. Eight of the indicators measuring care for chronic conditions relate to diabetic patients. The calculation of the performance payment for each physician is rather complex taking into account the doctor's individual performance, the average performance of all doctor's per indicator and the target objectives which are set annually by the Haute Autorité de Santé (HAS, the public entity responsible for setting health care quality standards). The indicators are a mix of measures for procedural quality (e.g. number of HbA1c tests) and intermediate outcomes (e.g. share of diabetics below HbA1c thresholds). They also include cholesterol thresholds and indicators to measure the intake of statins and aspirin among diabetics at high risk of developing cardiovascular diseases (CNAMTS, 2014; Cashin et al., 2014). The bonus payments GPs can generate through the ROSP accounted for 4.1% of total GP payment in 2014 (Rapport de la Commission des comptes de la sécurité sociale, 2015). In 2015, the average bonus was around EUR 6 800 (CNAMTS, 2016).

An additional service for diabetics called "SOPHIA" was been put in place in 2009. SOPHIA provides diabetes counselling and education by nurses over the phone employed by the statutory health insurance. GPs are also financially rewarded for submitting a completed medical questionnaire to health insurance funds for each patient registering for this service.

In Germany, improved diabetes care is incentivised through some of the DMPs which have been gradually introduced since 2002. The aim of the introduction of the DMPs was to improve the care process and the quality of medical care for people with chronic conditions. Currently, DMPs exist for six conditions including diabetes type 1, diabetes type 2, breast cancer, chronic obstructive pulmonary disease (COPD), asthma and coronary heart disease. DMPs are developed by the statutory health insurance funds and the regional organisations of statutory health insurance physicians following the guidelines set out by the Federal Joint Committee (G-BA) and need to be accredited by the Federal Insurance Agency (BVA). The type 2 diabetes DMP is by far the biggest DMP with 1 717 accredited programmes/contracts and nearly four million enrolled diabetic patients (BVA, 2015). The high number of DMP contracts is due to the high number of Health Insurance Funds and because DMP contracting is predominantly a regional matter. The participation of physicians and patients is voluntary.

Overall, there appears to be little variation with regards to the aim and content between the numerous DMP contracts within one clinical area. In practice, the DMP contracts are negotiated between Statutory Health Insurance Funds and regional associations of SHI-ffiliated doctors and define the tasks and responsibilities of physicians as well as stipulate the additional payments they can receive. The nature and the tariffs of these additional payments ultimately depend on the specific diabetes DMP contract but generally

GPs are paid for documentation and co-ordination of care, training and patient education. Physicians are only rewarded for fully documented patient files. This requires them to perform or initiate a number of services quarterly or annually.

In some cases, the DMP contracts can also stipulate a quality-related bonus such as in a DMP contract for the state of Thuringia where GPs can receive an additional payment if the share of diabetic patients that meet the Hb1Ac levels in their practice is above the benchmark value of their peers in the region.

2.4. Assessment of policy impact of add-on payments

This section assesses the payment reform in select countries by looking at whether policy objectives were met (such as achieving quality gains and/or savings) and highlights the conditions for implementation that either encouraged or hindered implementation (such as stakeholder engagement, administrative burden). This section follows the analytical framework applied to payment innovations throughout this report (Table 2.5), as a prism through which to assess the impact of the payment reform against the intended policy objective, across dimensions of quality, savings and unintended consequences, and considering conditions for implementation of the payment reform.

Add-on payments have been used widely, and are in place in many countries and across numerous domains of care. Available evidence suggests that add-on payments to promote care co-ordination have been relatively simple to implement, generally require modest IT requirements and data exchanges compared to the more sophisticated payment innovations. The add-on payments in France and Germany (discussed in Section 2.2) seem to show some positive results for selected quality indicators, though it can be difficult to separate their contribution to wider policy objectives, as well as to disentangle their "own" effects from the influence of other factors.

P4P for quality of care paid for ex post is increasingly being used in many countries, and across a growing diversity of settings. There have been recent shifts towards using outcome information and patient experience for payment, and countries with richer data infrastructures have greater scope to develop more sophisticated indicators. P4P programmes are commonly focussed on improving quality, and to some extent efficiency. P4P programmes have been associated with improvements in quality indicators, but it is yet unclear to what extent they are effective in improving health outcomes. Evidence of the impact of P4P programmes on costs is again limited and also depends on how the programmes are set up, notably whether they are conceived as budget neutral or whether new funds are made available. Hence, for some programmes there have been additional costs associated with implementing P4P. Despite the limited evidence on impact of P4Ps on health outcomes, efficiency and cost, their continued popularity among OECD countries may also reflect interest among policy makers to consider the broader health system effects such as an improvement in health data infrastructure, data availability or a greater focus on quality.

Table 2.5. Assessment of payment reform in select OECD countries

	Germany	France	Ontaorio, Canada	Portugal	Norway
Type and name of payment reform	Add-on co-ordination (Cardio-Integral)	Add-on co-ordination (ENMR)	Add-on payment (P4P) for some GP practices	Add-on payment (P4P) in primary care	Add-on payment (P4P) in hospitals
Assessment of policy impact					
Achievement in terms of policy objective					
Quality	+	+	+/-	+	evaluation due later
Savings	+	+		+	evaluation due later
Unintended consequences					
Conditions for implementation					
Payment reform embedded in larger policy reform	+	+	+	+	-
Stakeholder participation in policy development (e.g. actively consulted in establishment of law/scheme)			+	+	+
Payer participation	voluntary for SHI funds	mandatory payments by SHI	GPs choose from variety of organising models, some including P4P	dependent on provider take up	applied to all hospital regions
Provider participation	voluntary	voluntary	voluntary	voluntary	mandatory
Administrative burden					
Data collection and use			existing data	new data and existing	existing data
How are tariffs set	negotatiated by SHI funds and providers	individual tariff depend on staff size of setting and number of patients, the total amount available for ENMR set at national level	add-on payment for which eligibility varies between GP practice model	add-on payment based on nationally established indicators, and negotiated bonuses with local commissioner	around 0.5% of the block grant budget allocated to the (4) regional hospital associations is allocated through the P4P scheme
Independent evaluation of reform	+	+	-	+/-	- (forthcoming)

Source: Authors' compilation.

No clear breakthrough in performance improvement following the introduction of a P4P scheme can be identified

The popularity of P4P schemes in OECD countries continues to grow in primary care, specialist care as well as in hospitals, although there is still a scarcity of clear evidence on the success – or otherwise – of P4P programmes. Systematic reviews of available evidence tentatively suggest a positive impact on performance, but evidence on the impact of P4P on health outcomes remains inconclusive and limited. While improvements on some indicators in some P4P schemes are found, no clear "breakthrough" in performance improvement can be clearly linked to the introduction of a P4P scheme.

In Portugal, the reform to primary care, in which a P4P component was introduced, has shown improvements in care quality, patient and practitioner satisfaction (Lourenço, 2016; Lopes Ferreira and Raposo, 2015) but it is too early to determine whether these short-term improvements are sustainable in the long run (Perelman and Lourenço, 2015). The share of hypertensive patients with controlled blood pressure is significantly higher in FHU models A (53.8%) and B (where there is the greatest P4P component) (65.2%) than in traditional health care centres (37.8%). The same is true for controlled diabetics (Lourenço, 2016) (see Table 2.6).

In 2015, a EUROPEP[4] survey, which measures patient satisfaction, was carried out in a sample of primary care institutions in Portugal (Lopes Ferreira and Raposo, 2015). The survey covered traditional primary health care centres, FHU A and FHU B. Results showed that satisfaction with FHUs is good: on average, 76.6% of users of traditional centres would recommend the health facility to a friend, compared to 85.8% of FHU A users and 91.3% of FHU B users. The global level of patient satisfaction was highest for FHU B (79.5% of patients), followed by FHU Model A (76.8%) and traditional primary care centres (72.7%).

Table 2.6. Comparison of outcomes between traditional primary health care centres and Family Health Units in Portugal, 2013

	Traditional primary health care centres	FHU Model A	FHU Model B (with P4P component)
Proportion of controlled diabetics	41.5%	61.6%	70.3%
Proportion of hypertensive patients with controlled blood pressure	37.8%	53.8%	65.2%

FHU: Family Health Unit.

Source: Lourenço (2016).

Nonetheless, in Portugal as in other voluntary P4P schemes, the influence of self-selection should not be discounted. It is difficult to control for the fact that those providers who sign up for a voluntary scheme may already be performing better, and simply get paid for what they are doing anyway, and would show better performance on selected indicators regardless of whether there was a payment incentive. This effect could be more pronounced in the case of Portugal, where providers are expected to demonstrate a certain level of achievement on performance indicators before they can progress from Model A to Model B.

In Ontario, Canada P4P appears to be a popular complementary payment element for GP practices where it is an aspect of various new payment models. While selection into these models is voluntary, uptake has been good. P4P is normally tied to certain practice and staffing requirements, for instance patient registration goals, minimum staffing levels for group practices, and requirements for after-hours care delivery (Henry et al., 2012).

In Germany, there is some modest positive impact of the diabetes DMP on health care quality in a number of instances showing improved processes of care and better patient outcomes (Cashin et al., 2014). The DMPs were associated with improvement in the implementation of practice guidelines and a reduction of hospitalisation rates and mortality (Miksch et al., 2010; Drabik et al., 2012). Patients participating in the DMPs are more likely to receive structured and co-ordinated care than similar patients not enrolled in a DMP (Szecsenyi et al., 2008). These findings may also partially be explainable by self-selection of patients, with DMPs attracting the more motivated diabetic patients.

In Australia and France, results are mixed. In Australia, evidence is inconclusive as to whether the PIP leads to an increase in diabetic testing. Some positive impact on the completion of treatment cycles could be observed but was not controlled for underlying trends (Australian National Audit Office, 2010). Evaluation of the CAPI in France showed an increase in the number of doctors providing appropriate diabetes management but this difference was not significantly different from increases in the rate of doctors not participating in CAPI. More recent evaluations of the impact of the ROSP (which replaced CAPI) show improvement in the share of controlled diabetics with HbA1c values below 8.5% and also additional progress in relevant process indicators (e.g. the share of diabetic patients with three or four HbA1c test per year) (CNAMTS, 2016). However, given that the ROSP includes nearly all GPs, the influence of any trend effects cannot be distinguished from the impact of the ROSP incentives.

The case studies examined here, taken from Australia, Canada, France, Germany, Norway and Portugal, suggest some possible positive influence of P4P schemes on provider performance, in particular quality of care. However, no clear breakthrough in performance improvement following the introduction of a P4P scheme can be identified. When improvements in performance on collected indicators have been identified, it has been very difficult to separate out the influence of the change in payment method from other factors, such as the influence of self-selection (in Ontario, Canada and Portugal), underlying trends in improving quality of care (in Australia or France), or indeed changes or improvement to the way that relevant data is recorded and reported.

This finding is consistent with the findings of numerous systematic reviews of P4P programmes. Rosenthal and Frank (2006) conclude that "despite the assertions of its proponents, the empirical foundations of pay for performance in health care are rather weak", while Christianson et al. (2007) find that the strongest controlled studies provide little evidence that financial incentives improved quality of care. When quality improvements are identified, systematic reviews have, again similar to conclusions from case studies discussed here, found it difficult to disentangle to what degree they can be attributed to the change in payment (Petersen et al., 2006; Christianson et al., 2007). Where some positive outcomes following introduction of P4P have been identified, they have typically been mixed. Results have been found to vary across different areas of performance, for instance with positive results for clinical effectiveness and care equity but apparently less impact on co-ordination or continuity (Van Herck, 2010).

In a review of 12 P4P programmes, amongst them large and well-established programmes such as the United Kingdom's Quality and Outcomes Framework (QOF), the Australian PIP and French ROSP/CAPI, and three programmes from the United States concluded that the impact of P4P has been relatively minimal, even disappointing: "In common with many other authors, we too find that P4P has not produced the direct significant change in performance that many advocates hoped for" (Cashin et al., 2014, p. 15). The authors do find, though, that introduction of P4P programmes has brought some other important system benefits, amongst them clarification of the goals of providers, improved purchasing processes, better measurement of provider activity and performance, and more informed dialogue between purchasers and providers. In the English QOF, one of the most established P4P programmes which is voluntarily applied to GPs working for the NHS, a number of studies show high initial improvements in process indicators after introduction with little change since. Furthermore, little impact on health system performance beyond the immediate GP-provided care was seen, for instance lower hospital admission rates – which might be anticipated with improved primary care management – or an impact on mortality, could not be observed (Eijkenaar et al., 2013).

P4P can be an adaptable and versatile way to target and prioritise quality improvement

One of the strengths of P4P as an add-on payment is its versatility across care settings, with P4P programmes having been introduced to primary, outpatient specialist, and hospital care across a number of OECD countries.

Additionally, the shape of P4P systems is adaptable to system needs and policy priorities – within the constraints of available data. This adaptability has meant that, latterly, patient satisfaction has been introduced to P4P programme indicators in countries where such data is available, including Norway and Portugal. Though P4P programmes have most commonly focussed on intermediate outcome indicators, in Norway where cancer survival indicators for hospital were available and deemed appropriate, these outcome indicators have been used.

P4P programmes can be used to channel existing resources with attention to quality, and need not always demand significant investment of additional resources

Some P4P schemes have been introduced with significant injections of new funds, notably the UK QOF and Turkey's "Family medicine performance based contracting" scheme (Cashin et al., 2014). Others, including in Canada, Norway and Portugal, have for the most part sought to redistribute or redirect existing resources. In Portugal, the organisational and payment reforms which introduced P4P to primary care appear to have shown quality improvements, and some cost saving as unit costs per medical consultations are lower than in traditional health centres (Lourenço, 2016). Some schemes have a cap on the amount of performance-based rewards available, for instance in Norway where a fixed amount is distributed unequally between the four hospital regions based on their relative performance. In Ontario, Canada an estimated CAD 1.5 billion was invested in primary care, much of this devoted to developing alternative primary care models and alternative modes of payment (Sweetman and Buckley, 2014). Payment to physicians has been increasing at a faster rate than inflation, and much more rapidly than in the non-health workforce (Henry et al., 2012; Leonard and Sweetman, 2014).

In a system like the United Kingdom's QOF, where all performance points that are achieved are rewarded, performance-based payment is harder to anticipate and can be variable. Nonetheless, investment in design, introduction, and operation of P4P schemes is likely to incur at least initial additional costs. P4Ps schemes are typically associated with higher costs for the health systems including costs for the incentive, for administration and data verification as well as governance (Cashin et al., 2014).

That being said, in some instances improved care processes and efficiency gains led to system-wide savings such as the German DMP for chronic patients (including diabetes patients) in primary care and the Maryland Hospital Acquired Conditions Programme focussing on avoiding complications in the hospital sector (Cashin et al., 2014). Nonetheless, to date there is no clear evidence of P4P programmes that have been cost saving but it has to be borne in mind that in many countries the introduction of P4Ps aim at quality improvements where the generation of savings is a secondary objective at most.

Even when results suggest that P4P schemes are effective it is difficult to attribute successes to payment reform alone

Given a shortage of comprehensive evaluations of P4P schemes, it remains difficult to establish both to what extent P4P schemes are effective at improving quality of care, and to what extent they represent value for money.

The impact of P4P is very difficult to disentangle from other changes likely to influence the quality of care. In instances where P4P programmes are implemented alongside non-financial incentives such as performance feedback or public reporting, some of the potential performance improvement may be attributable to the alternative incentives (Eijkenaar et al., 2013). In some examples, it appears that other non-financial changes were at least as important as the payment mechanism change. For example, there are notable improvements in the quality of care in the new FHUs in Portugal, where P4P is a significant component of payment, but the payment reform was accompanied by significant organisational change. Indeed in Portugal, while a 2015 patient survey found higher overall levels of satisfaction with the primary care units which included a P4P payment component (FHU Model B), the same survey also showed that larger units showed higher levels of satisfaction regardless of the management model followed, and that the time since the establishment of the unit also positively influenced satisfaction. Even if areas targeted by P4P are showing improvements, these improvements might need to be seen in context of other broader dimensions, such organisational change in Portugal and Canada, and a broader reform agenda aimed at improving quality of care in Norway, for example.

2.5. Conditions for the implementation of P4P add-ons across health systems and care settings

Conditions for the implementation of P4P add-ons varied across health systems and care settings, but appear to include some broad pre-requisites for success. While a clear verdict on the overall success or otherwise of P4P programmes is hindered by patchy and incomplete evaluation, features of more successful P4P appear to include the use of measures where there is clear room for providers to improve performance, targeting individual physicians or small groups instead of large groups of providers, and rewarding absolute instead of relative targets (Eijkenaar et al., 2013; Cashin et al., 2014).

Stakeholder participation in the selection of indicators, a robust and sufficiently comprehensive source of data from which to develop indicators appears to have a broadly positive impact on the success of the introduction of P4P programmes. Even when a broad range of indicators are available for use in a P4P programme, it can be a challenge to identify the most effective indicators.

Despite the clear and apparently growing popularity of P4P payments, independent evaluations of reforms are not consistently undertaken; rigorous assessment following the introduction of P4P would help individual countries and systems understand what is working or not, and would contribute towards a deeper understanding of the broader trend.

P4P payments have been embedded in broader reforms to payment and organisation, and can be an important incentive for providers

In Norway, as well as in programmes such as the UK's QOF for primary care, the ROSP/CAPI for general practitioners in France, in the schemes introduced in primary care in Australia and New Zealand, and for hospitals in Korea and Maryland, United States (Cashin et al., 2014), P4P was introduced as an additional "add-on" payment (or penalty) without significant changes to the underlying organisational or payment model, with the objective to improve quality of care. That said, the introduction of P4P in Norway came as part of a broader reform on systematic quality improvement, as has been the case in other countries, for instance the UK's Quality Outcomes Framework (QOF). In other cases, though, accessing performance-based rewards has been conditional upon agreeing to other organisational or financial changes (meeting certain pre-requisites around quality of information or indicators). In Portugal, for instance, P4P was introduced to newly created primary care models. P4P was not introduced as an additional component to an existing payment model, but rather was part of a broader organisational change to primary care, and a shift from facility-level payment based on salaries to mixed payment including salary, capitation and P4P. This holds also true for Ontario, Canada where the P4P schemes introduced for primary care physicians were been tied closely to organisational changes, notably requirements that physicians work in group models, and that after-hours care be provided.

In both Portugal and Ontario the primary care re-organisation to which P4P is attached was voluntary for primary care practitioners, and appears to have had a good degree of success with quick up-take by practitioners, especially in Portugal.

Stakeholder participation has shown to have broad involvement

In two of the cases examined as part of this study, stakeholder participation in policy development had broad involvement and may well have had an indirect positive effect. In Norway there was broad involvement of key stakeholders, while in Portugal the initiative started as a pilot in 2005 where the Family Medicine Association and Medical Trade Unions were involved from the beginning as part of a broader primary care reform and improvement efforts before being scaled up. Stakeholder involvement was found to be important in ten out of the twelve P4P schemes (Cashin et al., 2014). Korea and Turkey were two exceptions.

In Estonia's scheme (Primary health care quality bonus scheme) for example, the Society of Family Doctors selected the performance indicators used in the scheme, while the Estonia Health Insurance Fund provided recommendations for implementation. In Brazil's Sao Paulo OSS, an Independent Assessment Commission made up of representatives of government and civil society reviewed performance indicators and calculated penalties. Involvement of broad stakeholders (such as academic experts and clinicians) through the National Institute for Health and Clinical Excellence (NICE) in the UK's QOF is seen as contributing to what is now a highly transparent and participatory process (Lester and Campbell, 2010). Following each revision to the QOF indicators, the proposed new indicators are made available for review through an open consultative process, following which final selections are made.

Stakeholder involvement in developing P4P programmes is judged by Cashin et al. (2014) to be an important part of aligning objectives, for instance between the government and health providers, for services, and thereby strengthening governance processes. Stakeholder participation, consultation and preferably buy-in appears to have a positive potential to support the success of a new scheme, while a failure to ensure stakeholder involvement may have damaging consequences.

Most P4P have been using process indicators or intermediate outcome indicators, with a more limited number of P4P programmes including patient experience measures

Policy objectives of P4P schemes differ between countries and can be wide ranging (quality, efficiency, access, improved outcomes). Policy objectives are influenced by the health priorities identified, the care setting (primary/specialist/hospital), as well as the choice of available indicators to measure performance.

Indicators which measure different domains of provider performance and quality are selected for P4P programmes in line with the objectives of the programme. Typical domains measured by these indicators include processes (e.g. the delivery of certain services, or timely treatment in certain domains), efficiency (e.g. expenditure on pharmaceuticals or generic drugs), and access (e.g. number of consultations per patient, or number of consultations by target patient group). Indicators of quality also include outcome indicators, mainly intermediate outcomes (for instance controlled blood pressure or Hba1C level). Of the programmes presented in this chapter, only Norway's hospital-based P4P programme includes non-intermediate outcome measures, notably cancer mortality.

Changes to the indicators used in P4P schemes can reflect changing policy priority, as well as adjustments to try to increase the impact of the P4P payment on performance. For instance, the well-established QOF programme in the United Kingdom sees indicators revised on an annual basis. Indicators are retired, for example, when the majority of GP practices are consistently performing in the upper quintiles, or if stakeholders involved in indicator selection consider that more effective measures are available. Differing approaches to the QOF indicators are used. Compared to other devolved nations in the United Kingdom, the number of indicators used and points attributed to the clinical domain was reduced in Wales, and eventually points in the clinical domain were removed completely for the 2015/16 QOF indicator set (OECD, 2016). This decision was taken because it was felt that the clinical indicators either had consistently high levels of performance achieved (for example heart disease area), and/or quality improvement work was ongoing or continuing through other channels. The removal of the clinical indicators was also part of a deliberate decision to use other policy tools to focus on professional clinical judgement – notably the use of best practice guidelines.

In primary care, process indicators are common, alongside a few intermediate outcome measures. Performance indicators in primary care cover different domains. The indicators used in FHUs in Portugal and in primary care in Ontario, Canada, are in large part focussed on clinical processes, and incentivising care that is consistent with best practice guidelines, but also cover access and efficiency domains (see Box 2.2). In Portugal, for example, the performance of each FHU is assessed with 22 indicators of which 10 can be negotiated between FHU and regional health authorities and 12 are common to all FHU (Lourenço, 2016). The indicators cover the full spectrum of the medical field, including family planning, child health, chronic diseases and mental health. Indicators related to clinical performance and efficiency have the biggest weight in the performance mix which determines the monetary bonus.

Box 2.2. Indicators used in add-on for primary care-based quality programmes in Canada and Portugal

In Ontario, Canada, all primary care incentives/bonuses available for general practitioners are process-based (none are outcome-based). Eligibility for the different incentives depends on the organising model that the GP practice is in; for instance, GPs under the Comprehensive Care Model are eligible for quite a few additional incentives, while GPs who are part of the Rural and Northern Physician Group Agreement are eligible for almost all incentives. Some incentives are more closely aligned to FFS add-ons or add-ons for co-ordination, e.g. bonus for providing smoking cessation, for managing a patient's diabetes, or for providing certain services such as home visits. Others are more typical of P4P programme incentives, and more similar to those seen in Portugal and Norway, for instance bonuses for immunising 60-80% of registered seniors.

In Portugal, for Model A and B FHUs, 22 indicators were selected for the P4P component, from a national set of more than 100 indicators. Target levels were set based on national health objectives, population characteristics, good practices, and historical data. Indicators cover four domains which are established nationally: access (two indicators, jointly weighting 7.5%), clinical performance (seven indicators, weighting 26%), efficiency (two indicators accounting for 24%), perceived quality (one indicator, 5%). An additional four indicators are selected regionally (weight 15%), two by sector (weight 7.5%), and each FHU proposes four indicators according to their own improvement quality plan (weight 15%). The indicators categorised under the clinical performance categories are a mix of clinical process indicators, and intermediate outcome measures. The traditional primary care models also report similar sets of indicators. The national set of indicators common to all FHUs from 2014 to 2016 is the following:

Box 2.2. Indicators used in add-on for primary care-based quality programmes in Canada and Portugal *(cont.)*

Indicator	Area	Type	Weight	ID
Proportion of patients with at least one medical appointment during the last three years	Horizontal	Access	4.50%	6
Rate of nursing home visits per 1 000 patients	Horizontal	Access	3.00%	4
Proportion of pregnant women with adequate follow-up	Women Health	Clinical Performance (process)	4.50%	51
Proportion of women in reproductive age with appropriate monitoring in family planning	Women Health/ Family planning	Clinical Performance (process)	5.00%	52
Proportion of Infants within the first year of life with adequate follow-up	New-born, child and adolescent care	Clinical Performance (process)	6.00%	58
Proportion of seniors without prescription anxiolytics, sedatives and hypnotics	Mental Health	Clinical Performance (intermediate outcome)	2.00%	56
Proportion of patients of more than 13 years old characterised with smoking habits in the last three years	Horizontal	Clinical Performance (process)	2.50%	47
Proportion of hypertensive patients younger than 65 years old with controlled blood pressure	Chronic diseases - High blood pressure	Clinical Performance (intermediate outcome)	3.00%	20
Proportion of controlled diabetics (HgbA1c <= 8.0 %)	Chronic diseases - Diabetes	Clinical Performance (intermediate outcome)	3.00%	39
Pharmaceuticals expenditure per user	Horizontal	Efficiency	16.00%	70
Ancillary exams expenditure per user	Horizontal	Efficiency	8.00%	71
Proportion of patients satisfied and very satisfied	Horizontal	Perceived quality	5.00%	72

Source: Henry et al. (2012) ; Lourenço (2016).

Where outcomes measures are included outside of hospital settings, they measure intermediate outcomes – controlled blood pressure, blood sugar, cholesterol – for instance in the California IHA programme or the QOF in the United Kingdom, and in the Portuguese FHUs. A recent scheme introduced in the state of Hidalgo (Mexico) for primary and hospital care also covers a wide range of performance indicators (Box 2.3).

Box 2.3. Results-based financing to increase effective coverage funded by Mexico's Seguro Popular: A case study from the state of Hidalgo

The introduction of public health insurance in Mexico ("Seguro Popular") in 2002 has contributed towards universal financial risk protection. However, effective coverage is low for chronic diseases, with only 26% and 30% of adult men and women, respectively, having access to preventive care. To address this challenge, the state of Hidalgo's Seguro Popular designed a results-based financial incentive scheme in 2014 to improve performance of key service outputs and health outcomes.

Providers are to receive an annual bonus or deduction on expected Seguro Popular subsidies based on their performance for 20 primary care and five hospital care indicators including diabetes, cardiovascular health, prenatal care, breast cancer screening, oral health, family planning, chronic disease prevention, reduction of preventable surgery and hospital readmissions.

Indicators were designed based on the best evidence of likely health impact, on the feasibility of implementing the scheme and monitoring provider performance. Baselines for each indicator were measured using surveys and other sources of data. Annual performance targets were defined using an expert panel to assess the provider's capacity to increase performance based on their degree of control over resources and outcomes.

The size of the incentive fund was estimated at 10% of the payer's budget. The monitoring system was designed to make use of existing information and information systems in accessible formats.

Source: González Block (2014).

When they are used, outcome measures – such as mortality – are typically confined to hospital settings. Norway's use of outcome indicators (cancer survival) is an interesting departure from typical P4P indicators, even for P4P schemes in hospitals (Box 2.4). Indeed the Norwegian QBF is quite unique, amongst these schemes but also amongst other schemes covered in recent OECD work (see Cashin et al., 2014; OECD, 2010), in that outcome indicators are included, and make up a significant proportion of performance incentives (50%).

Patient experience is an important outcome indicator of quality and a potential lever for quality improvement. Portugal and Norway, as well as England, Israel and Korea, have used patient experience measures in P4P schemes. They are also included as a tool for quality control in the Medicare ACO contracts in the United States (see Chapter 4).

Box 2.4. Indicators used in add-on for a hospital-based quality programme in Norway

In Norway's QBF programme, indicators are selected across three domains: outcome (50%), process (20%) and patient satisfaction (30%). Most of the indicators are measured at the hospital level, with only five-year survival rates for cancer measured on the regional level. Overall performance of hospital regions is calculated combining scores on all indicators across each of the domains and taking into account reporting quality, minimum performance levels, best performance (between hospital regions) and relative improvements in performance. The indicators measuring patient satisfaction come from the National Patient Satisfaction Survey which is developed by and conducted by the Norwegian Knowledge Centre.

In 2014 the indicators used were as follows:

10 Outcome indicators	13 Process indicators	10 Patient satisfaction
50 % (50 000 points)	**20 % (20 000 points)**	**30 % (30 000 points)**
Perineal tear, 3rd & 4th degree	Corridor patients	Information
Five-year survival rate for colon cancer, per health region	Discharge summary sent within 7 days	Nursing staff
Five-year survival rate for rectal cancer, per health region	Hip fracture operations performed within 48 hours	Physicians
Five-year survival rate for lung cancer, per health region	Postponement of planned operations	Organisation
Five-year survival rate for breast cancer, per health region	Thrombolysis treatments	Relatives
Five-year survival rate for prostate cancer, per health region	Initiated treatment of colon cancer within 20 days	Standard
30-day survival after hospital admission for hip fracture	Initiated treatment of lung cancer within 20 days	Discharge
30-day survival after hospital admission for myocardial infarction	Initiated treatment of breast cancer within 20 days	Co-ordination
30-day survival after hospital admission for stroke	Waiting time violations	Patient safety
30-day survival after hospital admission for all admissions	Registration of main diagnosis (Psychiatric care)	Waiting time
	Registration of main diagnosis (Addiction care)	
	Discharge summary sent within 7 days (Psychiatric care)	
	Discharge summary sent within 7 days (Addiction care)	

Source: Beck Olsen and Brandborg (2016).

The indicator choices for P4P add-ons vary between countries, even when the disease focus and care setting are the same

As described earlier, P4P schemes frequently target care for diabetes patients, but do not take the same approach in programme design, or in indicator selection.

In Australia, for instance, there are three different financial incentives in places in the framework of the Practice Incentive Program (PIP) to improve quality of diabetes care for type 2 patients. One component – the SIP – is targeted at the individual physician. The SIP can be claimed by GPs for each cycle of care completed for patients with diabetes. A cycle needs to be completed over a period of at least 11 months and up to 13 months. The SIP defines minimum requirements for 13 activities that need to be met under a cycle of care (Table 2.7).

Table 2.7. Performance indicators used in Australia's SIP programme targeting diabetes care

Activity	Frequency and description
Assess diabetes control by measuring HbA1c	At least once
Carry out a comprehensive eye examination	The patient must have had at least one comprehensive eye examination over the current and previous cycle of care
Measure weight and height and calculate Body Mass Index (BMI)	Measure height and weight and calculate the BMI on the patient's first visit and weigh them at least twice more
Measure blood pressure	At least twice
Examine feet	At least twice
Measure total cholesterol, triglycerides and HDL cholesterol	At least once
Test for micro albuminuria	At least once
Measure of the rate of the patient's expected Glomerular Filtration Rate (eGFR)	At least once
Provides self-care education	Provide patient education about diabetes management
Review diet	Review patient's diet and give them information on appropriate dietary choices
Review levels of physical activity	Review the patient's physical activity and give them information on appropriate levels of physical activity
Check smoking status	Encourage patient to stop smoking.
Review medication	Review patient's medication
Activities needed to be performed twice in a cycle of care must be performed at least five months apart	

Source: Department of Human Services (2013), "Practice Incentives Program, Diabetes Incentive Guidelines", Australian Government.

In France, high-quality diabetic care is also incentivised as part of the ROSP scheme; eight of the indicators measuring care for chronic conditions relate to diabetic patients (see Table 2.8). In Germany, due to differences in the arrangement of DMP diabetes contracts, there is more variety in the choice of activities targeted. Generally, GPs are rewarded for periodic documentation of treatment and the measurement of clinical indicators (HbA1c level) and bonuses are only paid for fully documented files. In that sense, it is similar to the Australian cycle of care. Additionally, patient education is an activity that can be rewarded. Recent trends in few regions show that relative performance in the share of patients with controlled HbA1c level are also used as performance indicators in some contracts (Kassenärztliche Vereinigung Thüringen, 2015).

In comparing the three diabetes P4P schemes some interesting differences emerge. Whereas in Australia and Germany, GPs receive rewards nearly exclusively for carrying out pre-defined activities (generally based on treatment guidelines) the focus in France lies more on the achievement of clinical indicators, such as the share of patients with diabetes with HbA1c levels below 8.5%. In the case of Australia, the P4P scheme provides patients with access to a range of pathology tests used in the diagnosis and management of diabetes. This includes HbA1c and other conventional tests, like oral glucose tolerance testing. It is up to the patient's treating practitioner to decide the testing regime that is appropriate to assist with patient management. The publicly subsidised pathology test items have service limits in line with clinical best practice. However, there is currently some discrepancy between peak practitioner groups on optimal testing intervals and this is the subject of review. The choice of indicators in France appears to indicate a focus of the ROSP on preventing complications. For patients with high blood pressure above a certain age, GPs are incentivised to prescribe low doses of aspirin to avoid cardiovascular complications.

Table 2.8. Indicators related to diabetes in the French ROSP

Domain	Category	Indicator	Intermediate objective	Target objective	Minimum threshold	Number of points	Equivalent in EUR	Type of indicator	Frequency
Chronic conditions	Diabetes	% of diabetic patients tested 3 or 4 times per year for HbA1c	54%	≥ 65%	10 patients	30	210	Calculated	Quarterly
		% of diabetic patients with HbA1c level < 8,5%	80%	≥ 90%	10 patients	15	105	Declared	Annually
		% of diabetic patients with HbA1c level < 7,5%	60%	≥ 80%	10 patients	25	175	Declared	Annually
		% of diabetic patients with LDL cholesterol level < 1,3 g/l	80%	≥ 90%	10 patients	10	70	Declared	Annually
		% of diabetic patients with LDL cholesterol level < 1,5 g/l	65%	≥ 80%	10 patients	25	175	Declared	Annually
		% of diabetic patients who had an eye exam in the past year	68%	≥ 80%	10 patients	35	245	Calculated	Quarterly
		% of diabetic patients treated with antihypertensive drug and statins among men > 50 years and women> 60 years	65%	≥ 75%	10 patients	35	245	Calculated	Quarterly
		% of diabetic patients treated with antihypertensive drug, statins and aspirin at low dose in diabetic patients treated with antihypertensive drug and statins	52%	≥ 65%	10 patients	35	245	Calculated	Quarterly

Source: CNAMTS – Caisse Nationale d'Assurance Maladie des Travailleurs Salariés (2015).

Absolute, relative and competitive targets are used across different P4P schemes, and also within single schemes. Popularity seems to vary, while both Eijkenaar (2013) and Cashin et al. (2014) suggest that absolute measures are preferred. Many countries have schemes that combine these different modes of target setting and these mixed schemes tend to be more common in specialist and acute hospital care. In Portugal, indicators are used to meet absolute target thresholds, while in Norway absolute and relative rankings are used.

A number of payment schemes use absolute measures (e.g. screening rate of 8%) to set a minimum standard, which is then supplemented with or sits alongside differently adjusted targets. In Portugal, the proportion of hypertensive patients with controlled blood pressure, and the proportion of controlled diabetics (HgbA1c <= 8.0%) are included as indicators, and similar absolute targets are used in the ROSP in France. In the case of the ROSP, the calculation of the performance payment for each physician is, however, complex, taking into account the doctor's individual performance, the average performance of all doctors' per indicator, and the target objectives which are set annually by the "Haute Autorité de Santé" (HAS). In Norway, for the indicator "Perineal tear 3rd and 4th degree", the target was 2.3% of all vaginal births in 2015. A region reporting a higher rate will not earn points for this indicator. The number of points available will be distributed equally between the regions who meet this minimum target.

The introduction of P4P schemes can motivate providers towards better and broader data collection

Unlike many P4P schemes, the examples of P4P programmes explored in this publication draw on existing data resources to develop indicators for rewarding performance. Norway and Portugal in particular have impressive and comprehensive health system information systems. In Portugal, the use of existing data sets has meant that both types of FHUs which include a P4P component, and the traditional primary care models report similar sets of indicators and can be more easily compared directly. In Norway, the use of a pre-existing data set, which already covers a number of years, has been a contributor to the inclusion of outcome indicators (cancer survival) in the scheme.

While in Norway and Portugal pre-existing rich data infrastructures have supported the introduction of P4P, it remains the case that in many countries good building blocks for P4P – notably appropriate performance measures – are missing. However, it is clear that the introduction of P4P programmes can bring significant incentives for improvements in data systems and reporting of data. Data improvements have come through direct incentives for providers to invest in information infrastructure (IT, electronic medical records) as in the Australian PIP, California's IHA, and France's ROSP/CAPI, or related to minimum IT standards being a criterion for participation in the P4P scheme, for instance in the UK QOF.

The collection of appropriate indicators for P4P schemes, and other add-on payments, needs to strike the right balance between targeting the most appropriate indicators, and the administrative burden data reporting imposes on providers and practitioners. If too narrow a selection of indicators is chosen, the risk is both of narrowing focus of the incentives, and of encouraging providers to disproportionally focus care provision on areas tied to the incentive payment (Eijkenaar, 2013; Cashin et al., 2014). On the other hand, a broader range of indicators, and a broader definition of performance, can contribute more comprehensively to improving performance, but a large number of indicators can lead to a more significant administrative burden, and mean that incentives become unclear. The data sources used in P4P programmes will also have an impact on administrative burden; if pre-existing data sources are used, as in Norway and Portugal, the introduction of incentives tied to the data is unlikely to entail new data reporting burdens, but may help improve reporting rate and fidelity.

Given that the P4P component is usually small, the dominant or co-existing payment systems remain influential

Given that the P4P component is usually small, the dominant or co-existing payment systems remain influential and their impact in relation to the P4P objectives has to be considered.

P4P incentives typically amount to less than 5% of total income/revenues with the QOF in England reporting around 15% (OECD Health Systems Characteristics Survey 2012), meaning that co-existing payment systems are – almost without exception – also the dominant payment system. Even in Portugal where P4P payments can amount to as much as 30% of overall revenues, other payment mechanisms account for a greater revenue share. In the hospital sector, the share is much smaller, for instance 0.5% in Norway, or up to 4% in the Portuguese performance-based contracting mechanism for public hospitals (OECD, 2014).

The dominant payment system has the potential to either undo the effects of P4P programmes, or reinforce them in instances where the goal of both incentive structures aligns (Van Herck et al., 2010). Despite all reported examples of P4P for health providers sitting alongside other payment mechanisms, research on the interaction between P4P and the dominant payment system is quite weak.

Negative penalties are being used in performance-based payment schemes in hospitals

The achievement of desired targets can result in supplementary payment or in negative financial penalties. Often, the penalty takes the form of a proportion of nominally attributed funds being withheld. This is the case in the hospital P4P scheme of Norway. The payment covered by the P4P programme is capped (approximately NOK 500 million), and covers a small part of the block grant each region receives annually. This payment is distributed between the regions based on their attainment of absolute performance targets, and their improvement relative to the other hospital regions. This means that some hospital regions see an increase in payment, while others see a decrease relative to previous years (see Table 2.9).

Table 2.9. Comparison of income effect for each Regional Hospital Association in 2015 under Norwegian P4P scheme ("Quality Based Financing")

Regional Hospital Association	Difference with how the block budget would be distributed if quality performance was not taken into account, compared to under the P4P scheme	Difference in percent
South-East	-21 187 811	-7.70%
West	7 936 991	8.20%
Central	7 602 096	10.40%
North	5 648 724	8.60%

Source: Beck Olsen and Brandborg (2016).

Since 2008, the Centres for Medicare and Medicaid Services (CMS) use similar negative incentives for hospital performance in the United States where payments can be withheld for certain avoidable conditions, including "never" events and other complications that were not present on admission such as hospital-acquired infections, or have been shown to be largely preventable (Nuffield Trust, 2012). From 2012, CMS introduced penalties for readmissions (hospitals only) following acute myocardial infarction, congestive heart failure and pneumonia. The "excessive readmission rates" includes adjustments for clinical factors such as patient demographic attributes, comorbidities, and patient "frailty". The hospital payment penalty was initially set at 1% of every Medicare payment for a hospital that was established as having excessive readmissions across the three conditions, a penalty which rose to 2% in 2013 and 3% in 2014. In 2015, additional conditions were added to the calculation of the readmissions ratio. Preliminary data on the impact of the penalties on avoidable readmissions shows a small reduction in readmissions; 30-day hospital readmission was around 19% between 2007 and 2011, and then dropped following the introduction of the penalty, to 18.5% in 2012 and slightly below 18% in 2013 (ACEP, 2015).

Independent evaluation of reform

There have not, to date, been comprehensive independent reforms of either the P4P programme in Canada or Norway.

In Portugal, several independent assessments have been undertaken. The Portuguese Court of Auditors carried out an audit from 2006 and 2012, which concluded that the FHU model shows, on average, greater economic efficiency, in the unit cost per medical consultation or user, when compared with traditional primary health care centres, which have higher unit costs. However, this audit was very controversial and almost all stakeholders contested its conclusions (Tribunal de Contas, 2014). Other studies found a systematic improvement in the quality indicators related to prevention, with less clear effects on access indicators and efficiency where further research is needed (Barros et al., 2015; Entitdade Reguladora Da Saúde, 2016).

In Portugal and Canada the existence of non-affiliated primary care physicians does give some scope for comparison of results. In Portugal, the Regional Health Authorities and the Central Administration for the Health System produce annual reports showing the results achieved by FHU and traditional primary health care centres. Invariably, FHU achieve better access to care, and clinical performance and higher efficiency. For example, recent data from 2013 show that hypertensive patients and diabetics are better controlled by USF than traditional health care centres. Nonetheless, in Portugal as in other voluntary P4P schemes, the influence of self-selection should not be discounted. It is difficult to control for the fact that those providers who sign up for a voluntary schemes may already be performing better, and simply get paid for what they are doing anyway, and would show better performance on selected indicators regardless of whether there was a payment incentive.

A full independent evaluation of the reforms discussed in this chapter and their impacts would be very valuable in each case. Such an evaluation is expected from Norway in the near future. As this chapter has pointed out, despite the increasing popularity of P4P programmes, clear evidence of their efficacy and impact is still very weak. A better understanding of the successes and failures of P4P as an approach, and individual P4P programmes, would be greatly advanced by more thorough independent evaluations of existing programmes. While independent evaluation of P4P reforms should be valuable, undertaking the evaluation can be complex. Given the introduction of P4P schemes as part of broader reform and focus on quality improvement may contribute to more significant improvements in quality, but it is extremely difficult to assess the extent to which broader reforms have multiplied the effect of P4P schemes, or indeed whether improvements would have been equivalent with or without either P4P introduction or other quality efforts. In the United Kingdom, for example, where evidence suggests that quality-related processes, and quality of care for chronic conditions improved following the introduction of the QOF, attribution of improvements to the QOF is difficult given that the trend towards improvement had already started, and given the lack of control group for comparison (Charlesworth et al., 2014).

Indeed, identifying a suitable comparison group to evaluate the P4P reform can be challenging. In the case studies examined in this chapter, the challenge is a clear consideration in Norway – where the application of the reform to all relevant providers means that no control group is available – and in Portugal where selection bias for providers is a clear consideration, given that primary care providers had to demonstrate sufficiently good performance even before they joined the P4P scheme, while peers under traditional payment models did not have to meet such performance benchmarks. Ideally, evaluations would highlight the isolated impact of the financial incentives associated with payment reform. This would require having control groups – providers that do not participate in the P4P programme (to identify overall trends in quality indicators) – and randomised participation among providers (to avoid self-selection), and to leave patients ignorant about participation of their clinicians (to avoid patient selection). In complex OECD health systems, where financing, governance, stakeholder views, and patient rights can be highly challenging to navigate, setting up such elaborated evaluations may be very difficult.

There is a need for more rigour in evaluation methods. In particular, clear considerations for evaluation, including what to evaluate, when to evaluate, the scope of evaluation, and the need to focus on the beneficiaries of P4P programmes (Cashin et al., 2014).

The question of "what" to evaluate is a challenge. Evaluation might consider performance against the intended goals of the payment reform, as this report does. In a scheme-specific evaluation, though, it is worth looking beyond targeted goals – and identified indicators – to consider spillover effects and unintended consequences. There is an understanding that P4P payments may encourage overprovision of unnecessary services covered by the scheme and thus need to be designed so they do not discourage non-incentivised activities (Flodgren et al., 2011; Scott et al., 2011; Sherry, 2015).

As Cashin et al. (2014) state, most impact evaluations are conducted based on the measures and indicators collected to calculate performance within the programme, but a major concern is that providers shift their efforts towards measured indicators or targeted patients at the expense of unmeasured areas. Equally, P4P programmes may well have positive spillover effects, such as positive impacts on quality of care in areas not reflected in measured indicators, or in increasing data availability or reporting rate. There is a clear case for evaluations to take a broader perspective on the impact of the performance.

2.6. Conclusion

Add-on payments have been used widely, and are in place in many countries and across numerous domains of care. Add-on payments to promote care co-ordination, where payments can be made both ex ante and ex post, have been relatively simple to implement. In most instances, there has been little provider resistance to their introduction, and they generally require fewer IT requirements and data exchanges compared to the more sophisticated payment innovations where payments rely on the measurement of patient metrics. They display some positive results for selected quality indicators in France and higher patient satisfaction in Germany and providers supported their introduction.

However, it can be difficult to separate their contribution to wider policy objectives, as well as to disentangle their "own" effects from the influence of other factors.

P4P or add-on payments for quality of care (where payment is made ex post) are increasingly being used in many countries; numbers of P4P schemes continue to increase across the OECD, and across different care settings. There have been recent shifts towards using outcome information and patient experience for payment, and countries with richer data infrastructures have greater scope to develop more sophisticated indicators. Quite often, P4P payments are small as share of provider income and therefore other co-existing payment mechanisms remain strongly influential. P4P policies in Portugal have shown some positive impact on quality and health system governance, especially when used in conjunction with broader organisational or financial reform, and while evaluations are pending in Norway, the ambitious programme is embedded in a quality improvement agenda, and could be reasonably expected to have a positive impact on directing greater attention to quality and outcomes. The inclusion of both patient satisfaction assessments and patient outcomes (cancer survival) is innovative, and a comprehensive assessment would likely be of great interest to policy makers, payers and providers across OECD countries. While P4P programmes are commonly focussed on improving quality, and to some extent efficiency, evidence of the impact of programmes on costs is again limited. Indeed, while for some programmes there have been additional costs associated with implementing P4P, there is no conclusive evidence of any P4P programme which has been cost saving.

Despite the limited evidence on the impact of P4Ps on outcomes, the continued popularity among OECD countries may also reflect interest among policy makers to consider the broader health system effects such as an improvement in health data infrastructure, data availability or a greater focus on quality in discussions between purchasers and providers.

P4P programmes continue to be introduced in OECD countries, with programmes planned or in early stages in the hospital sector for France and Germany, in Latvian primary care, and in Mexico across a range of providers. Given the now-significant range of add-on programmes for quality, in terms of country range, application across provider settings, and programme scale, comprehensive national evaluations of programmes are now needed in order to fully take stock of the successes and failures of P4P. Ideally, evaluations would highlight the isolated impact of the financial incentives associated with payment reform, an approach that would likely require double-blind control groups of patients and providers, but this would be most likely extremely difficult to introduce in reality. Nonetheless, this does not preclude the introduction of greater rigour in evaluation methods, and the systematic inclusion of evaluation mechanisms in payment reforms.

Notes

1. From an international perspective, waiting times for specialist treatment in Germany do not appear to be a major concern (The Commonwealth Fund, 2013).

2. The "Contrat d'amélioration des pratiques individuelles" (CAPI) targeting GPs was replaced by the "Rémunération sur objectifs de santé publique" (ROSP) in 2012, which also opened the scheme to outpatient specialists.

3. "Médecin traitant" can be loosely translated as "Primary physician". Patients can choose whether they have a "médecin traitant" or not, but face significantly lower reimbursements if they choose not to. The "médecin traitant" can be GP or specialist and their role is to guide patients through the health system and keep patients medical records. If patients have an attested long-term condition ("affection de longue durée") the "médecin traitant" receives an annual payment for documentation and co-ordination.

4. EUROPEP is a 23-item validated instrument and internationally standardised measure of patient evaluations of general practice care.

References

ACEP – American College of Emergency Physicians (2015), "Medicare's Hospital Readmission Reduction Program FAQ", American College of Emergency Physicians, http://www.acep.org/, accessed 01.08.2015.

Administração Central do Sistema de Saúde (2015), "Bilhete de Identidade dos Indicadores de Contratualização dos Cuidados de Saúde Primários no Ano de 2015", Administração Central do Sistema de Saúde, Lisboa, http://www.acss.min-saude.pt/Portals/0/bilhete_identidade_indicadores_contratualizacao_2015___2015_01_26.pdf.

Australian National Audit Office (2010), *Practice Incentives* Program, Department of Health and Ageing.

Barros, P.P. et al. (2015), "Políticas Públicas em Saúde: 2011-2014 Avaliação do Impacto [Public Health Policies 2011-2014; Impact Evaluation], Nova Healthcare Initiative – Research: 202, Lisboa, http://ppbarros.fe.unl.pt/My%20Shared%20Documents/Pol%C3%ADticas%20Públicas%20em%20Saúde%20(light).pdf.

Beck Olsen and Brandborg (2016), "Norway Case Example", submitted for the OECD Project on Payment Systems, http://www.oecd.org/health/paying-providers.htm.

Bundesversicherungsamt (2015), "Zulassung der strukturierten Behandlungsprogramme [Disease Management Programme – DMP] durch das Bundesversicherungsamt (BVA)", http://www.bundesversicherungsamt.de/weitere-themen/disease-management-programme/zulassung-disease-management-programme-dmp.html, accessed 28 Sept. 2015.

Cashin, C. et al. (2014), *Paying for Performance in Health Care: Implications for Health System Performance and Aaccountability*, European Observatory on Health Systems and Policies.

Charlesworth, A., L. Hawkins and L. Marshall (2014), "NHS Payment Reform: Lessons from the Past and Directions for the Future", Nuffield Trust, http://www.nuffieldtrust.org.uk/publications/nhs-payment-reform-lessons.

Christianson, J.B., S. Leatherman and K. Sutherland (2007), *Financial Incentives, Healthcare Providers and Quality Improvements: A Review of the Evidence*, The Health Foundation, London.

CMS – Centres for Medicare and Medicaid Services (2015), "Nursing Home Value-based Purchasing Demonstration – Factsheet", http://innovation.cms.gov/Files/fact-sheet/NHP4P-Fact-Sheet.pdf, accessed 7 Sept. 2015.

CNAMTS – Caisse Nationale d'Assurance Maladie des Travailleurs Salariés (2016), "La rémuneration sur objectifs de santé publique, quatre ans après. Point presse de l'assurance maladie 21/04/2016", Paris.

CNAMTS (2015), "Note méthodologique du dispositif de rémunération sur objectifs de santé publique des médecins traitants. Les indicateurs portant sur la qualité de la pratique médicale – Actualisation novembre 2015", Paris.

CNAMTS (2014), "La rémunération sur objectifs de santé publique, deux ans après. Point presse de l'assurance maladie 10/04/2014", Paris.

Commonwealth Fund (2015), *International Profiles of Health Care Systems 2014*, Washington.

Commonwealth Fund (2013), *2013 International Health Policy Survey in Eleven Countries*, Washington.

da Silva Fialho, A.S. (2008), "Family Health Units vs. Primary Health Care Centres. Development of Discrete Event Simulation Models to Compare the Performance of the Two Organizational Models", Instituto Superior Técnico, UTL, Lisbon.

Department of Health (2016a), "England Case Example – Smoking Cessation Programmes in England", unpublished, submitted to the OECD Project on Payment Systems.

Department of Health (2016b), "The Pharmaceutical Benefit Scheme – Sixth Community Pharmacy Agreement – Community pharmacy programmes", Australian Government, http://www.pbs.gov.au/info/general/sixth-cpa-pages/community-pharmacy-programmes.

Department of Human Services (2013), "Practice Incentives Program, Diabetes Incentive Guidelines –October 2013", Australian Government.

Drabik, A. et al. (2012), "Life Prolonging of Disease Management Programs in Patients with Type 2 Diabetes Is Cost-effective", *Diabetes Research and Clinical Practice*, Vol. 95, No. 2, pp. 194-200.

Eijkenaar, F. et al. (2013), "Effects of Pay for Performance in Health Care: A Systematic Review of Systematic Reviews", *Health Policy*, Vol. 110, pp. 115-130.

Entitdade Reguladora Da Saúde (2016), "Estudo sobre as unidades de saúde familiar e as unidades de cuidados de saúde personalizados" [Study of the family health units and the traditional primary care models], Entitdade Reguladora Da Saúde, Lisbon, https://www.ers.pt/uploads/writer_file/document/1793/ERS_-_Estudo_USF_e_UCSP_-_final__v.2_.pdf.

Flodgren, G. et al. (2011), "An Overview of Reviews Evaluating the Effectiveness of Financial Incentives in Changing Healthcare Professional Behaviours and Patient Outcomes", *Cochrane Database of Systematic Reviews*, Vol. 7, Art. No. CD009255, http://dx.doi.org/10.1002/14651858.CD009255.

González Block, M. (2014), *Estudio de caso de la compra estratégica del Seguro Popular* [Case study of strategic purchasing of Seguro Popular], Organización Panamericana de la Salud, Mexico City.

Henry, D. et al. (2012), "Payments to Ontario Physicians from Ministry of Health and Long-Term Care Sources 1992/93 to 2009/10 – ICES Investigative Report", ICES, Toronto, http://www.ices.on.ca/~/media/Files/Atlases-Reports/2012/Payments-to-Ontario-physicians-from-MOHLTC-sources/Full%20report.ashx.

IRDES (2014b), "L'évaluation de la performance des maisons, pôles et centres de santé dans le cadre des Expérimentations des nouveaux modes de rémunération (ENMR) sur la période 2009-2012", *Les Rapports de L'IRDES*, No. 559, December.

IRDES (2014a), "Les formes du regroupement pluriprofessional en soins de premier recours", *Questions d'économie de la Santé*, No. 201, September.

IRDES (2013), "The Impact of Multi-professional Group Practices on Healthcare Supply", *Questions d'économie de la Santé*, No. 189, July-August.

Kantarevic, J. and B. Kralj (2015), "Physician Payment Contracts in the Presence of Moral Hazard and Adverse Selection: The Theory and its Application to Ontario", *IZA Discussion Paper No. 9142*, Bonn, June

Kantarevic, J. and B. Kralj (2013), "Link between Pay for Performance Incentives and Physician Payment Mechanisms: Evidence from the Diabetes Management Incentive in Ontario", *Health Economics*, Vol. 22, pp. 1417-1439.

Kassenärztliche Vereinigung Thüringen (2015), "Vertrag über die Vergütung und Abrechnung von DMP-Leistungen für die Disease-Management-Programme vom 17.02.2014", http://www.kv-thueringen.de/mitglieder/dmp/02_verguetungsvertraege/01_vergue_ueberg_ohne-brust/01_verguetungsvertr.pdf, accessed 28 Sept. 2015.

Kiran, T. et al. (2014), "The Relationship between Primary Care Models and Processes of Diabetes Care in Ontario", *Canadian Journal of Diabetes*, Vol. 38, pp. 172-178.

Leonard, P.S.J. and A. Sweetman (2014), "Paying the Health Workforce", in Gregory P. Marchildon and Livio Di Matteo (eds.), *Bending the Cost Curve in Health Care: Canada's Provinces in International Perspective*, University of Toronto Press, Toronto, pp. 139-168.

Lester, H. and S. Campbell (2010), "Developing Quality and Outcomes Framework (QOF) Indicators and the Concept of 'QOFability'", *Quality in Primary Care*,Vol. 18, pp. 103-109.

Li, J. et al. (2013), "Physician Response to Pay-for-performance: Evidence from a Natural Experiment", *Health Economics*, Vol. 23, No. 8, pp. 962-978, August.

Lopes Ferreira, P. and V. Raposo (2015), "Monitorização da satisfação dos utilizadores das USF e de uma amostra de UCSP – Relatório Final", CEISUC, http://www.acss.min-saude.pt/Portals/0/2015.08.24-Relat%C3%B3rio%20Final-VF.pdf.

Lourenço, A. (2016), "Portugal Case Example on Primary Care", submitted for the OECD Project on Payment Systems, http://www.oecd.org/health/paying-providers.htm.

Marchildon, G.P. and B. Hutchison (2016), "Primary Care in Ontario, Canada: New Proposals after 15 Years of Reform", Health Reform Monitor, *Health Policy*.

McLeod, H. et al. (2015), "Effect of Pay-For-Outcomes and Encouraging New Providers on National Health Service Smoking Cessation Services in England: A Cluster Controlled Study", *PLoS ONE*, Vol. 10, No. 4, e0123349, http://dx.doi.org/10.1371/journal.pone.0123349.

Medicare Australia (2010), Audit Report No.5 2010-11, Performance Audit, Canberra.

Miksch, A. et al. (2010), "Is There a Survival Benefit within a German Primary Care-based Disease Management Program?, *American Journal of Managed Care*, Vol. 16, No. 1, pp. 49-54.

Milstein, R. and R. Blankart (2016), "German Case Example", submitted for the OECD Project on Payment Systems, http://www.oecd.org/health/paying-providers.htm.

Milstein, R. and J. Schreyögg (2015), "A Review of Pay-for-performance Programs in the Inpatient Sector in OECD Countries", Research Paper, Hamburg Center for Health Economics, No. 2015/09.

Ministère des Affaires Sociales, de la Santé et des Droits des Femmes (2015), "Communiqué de Presse – 20 février 2015", http://www.social-sante.gouv.fr/IMG/pdf/03_09_13_CP_PTMG.pdf.

Nuffield Trust (2012), *Reforming Payment for Health Care in Europe to Achieve Better Value*, Research Report, London.

OECD (2016), *OECD Reviews of Health Care Quality: United Kingdom 2015: Raising Standards*, OECD Publishing, Paris, http://dx.doi.org/10.1787/9789264239487-en.

OECD (2015), *OECD Reviews of Health Care Quality: Portugal 2015: Raising Standards*, OECD Publishing, Paris, http://dx.doi.org/10.1787/9789264225985-en.

OECD (2014), "Paying Providers for Health Care. Results of the 2012 Health Systems Characteristics Survey", data files at: http://www.oecd.org/els/health-systems/paying-providers.htm.

OECD (2012), "OECD Health Systems Characteristics Survey", Paris.

OECD (2010), *Value for Money in Health Spending*, OECD Publishing, Paris, http://dx.doi.org/10.1787/9789264088818-en.

Or, Z. and U. Häkinnen (2011), "DRGs and Quality: For Better or Worse?", in R. Busse, A. Geissler, W. Questin and M. Wiley (eds), *Diagnosis-related Groups in Europe – Moving Towards Transparency, Efficiency and Quality in Hospitals*, European Observatory on Health Systems and Policies Series.

Paris, V., M. Devaux and L. Wei (2010), "Health Systems Institutional Characteristics: A Survey of 29 OECD Countries", *OECD Health Working Papers*, No. 50, OECD Publishing, Paris, http://dx.doi.org/10.1787/5kmfxfq9qbnr-en.

Perelman, J. and A. Lourenço (2015), "Effectiveness of Pay-for-performance in Primary Care: The Portuguese Experience. 14ª Conferência Nacional de Economia da Saúde", Associação Portuguesa de Economia da Saúde, Lisboa, https://doc.co/SGWFE7/rHhfxc.

Petersen, L.A. et al. (2006), "Does Pay-for-Performance Improve the Quality of Health Care?", *Annals of Internal Medicine*, Vol. 145, pp. 265-272.

Rapport de la Commission des comptes de la sécurité sociale (2015), "Résultats 2014 Prévisions 2015", Paris, juin, Comptes de la sécurité sociale, http://www.securite-sociale.fr/IMG/pdf/rapport-ccss-20160120-114010-207-54.pdf.

Rosenthal, M.B. and R.G. Frank (2006), "What Is the Empirical Basis for Paying for Quality in Health Care?", *Medical Care Research and Review*, Vol. 63, pp. 135-157.

Royal Australian College of General Practitioners and Diabetes Australia (2014), "General Practice Management of Type 2 Diabetes – 2014-15", Melbourne.

Scott, A. et al. (2011), "The Effect of Financial Incentives on the Quality of Health Care Provided by Primary Care Physicians", *Cochrane Database of Systematic Reviews*, Vol. 9, Art. No. CD008451, http://dx.doi.org/10.1002/14651858.CD008451.pub2.

Sherry, T.B. (2015), "A Note on the Comparative Statics of Pay-for-Performance in Health Care", Health Economics, http://dx.doi.org/10.1002/hec.3169.

Sweetman, A. and G. Buckley (2016), "Canada Case Example (Ontario)", submitted for the OECD Project on Payment Systems, http://www.oecd.org/health/paying-providers.htm.

Sweetman, A. and G. Buckley (2014), "Ontario's Experiment with Primary Care Reform", School of Public Policy Research Paper, Vol. 7, No. 11, University of Calgary, pp. 1-35, http://www.policyschool.ucalgary.ca/?q=content/ontarios-experiment-primary-care-reform.

Szecsenyi, J. et al. (2008), "German Diabetes Disease Management Programs Are Appropriate for Restructuring Care According to the Chronic Care Model: An Evaluation with the Patient Assessment of Chronic Illness Care Instrument", *Diabetes Care*, Vol. 31, No. 6, pp. 1150-1154.

Tribunal de Contas (2014), "Audioria ao desempenho de unidades funcionais de cuidados de saúde primários" [Audit of the family health units in primary care], Tirbunal de Contas, Lisbon.

Van Herck, P. et al. (2010), "Systematic Review: Effects, Design Choices, and Context of Pay-for-performance in Health Care", *BMC Health Services Research*, Vol. 10:247.

Werblow, A. and A. Karman (2012), "Evaluation des Integrierten Versorgungsvertrages über die Versorgung kardiovaskulär erkrankter Versicherter (Cardio-Integral) der AOK Plus", http://www.aok-gesundheitspartner.de/imperia/md/gpp/sac/iv/vertraege/sac_cardio_integral_eva_endbericht.pdf.

Wong, C.Y. et al. (2016), "Consultancy on the Health Care Pathways, Provider Payment and Associated Costs of Patients with Diabetes", unpublished, submitted to the OECD Project on Payment Systems.

Chapter 3

Bundled health care provider payments

"Bundled" payments for health care, where several services relevant to a condition or intervention are grouped together for payment, are being used in several OECD countries. Bundled payments go beyond DRG payments, and aim to encourage cost savings and quality improvements for acute episodes of care such as elective surgical interventions and care for chronic conditions such as diabetes.

This chapter studies the policy impact of bundled payment in several OECD countries, including England (United Kingdom), Sweden, Portugal, the Netherlands, Denmark and the United States. The payment reform is assessed, with a particular focus on health care spending and quality. The discussion considers the policy goals, design of the payment reform, implementation process, and conditions for implementation, including IT requirements and stakeholder involvement.

3.1. Overview

"Bundled" payments for health care, where several services relevant to a condition or an intervention are grouped together for payment, are being used in several OECD countries. In this chapter the term bundled payments refers to innovations that group activities into a single tariff that go beyond simple DRG payments. They aim to encourage cost savings and quality improvements for acute episodes of care such as elective surgical interventions and care for chronic conditions such as diabetes.

Single payments for acute care episodes that bundle inpatient activities are not new. These DRG-type payments, which cover inpatient activities, have now been used for at least two decades in some OECD countries (see Chapter 1). They typically calculate tariffs based on average costs of care provision. Other more recent experiments in the United States have widened the scope of bundled payment, to include activities that occur before and after admission. In others, such as England and Sweden, quality is incorporated in the bundled payments through "best practice tariffs" or paying for outcomes, including surgical interventions for hip, knee and spine.

Chronic conditions, too, are being paid for through bundled payments, and push the scope of bundled payments beyond the inpatient sector. A policy focus on chronic conditions in part reflects a broader health policy objective of improving co-ordination of care. Indeed, patients with chronic conditions typically require the involvement of more than one health care provider. Separate payment systems for each provider reinforce fragmentation across the care pathway. Bundled payments for chronic conditions give shared incentives to providers across the chronic care pathway, and look to encourage a longer term emphasis on continued care, rather than one-off episodes or interventions.

This chapter considers these recent approaches to bundled payments, for episodic care and for chronic conditions, taking several case studies from OECD countries including England, Sweden, Portugal, the Netherlands, Denmark and the United States. All examples presented in the chapter have been rolled out or at least piloted. The only exception is the bundled payment for Parkinson's disease in the Netherlands which is currently still in a planning phase. The chapter starts by describing the key characteristics of these payment reforms, and then assesses their impact, including conditions for implementation. Finally, the discussion sets out key building blocks to implement a bundled payment followed by concluding remarks.

3.2. Episode-based payments incentivising best practice or improvement of patient outcomes

Bundled payments have a number of characteristics (see Table 3.1). The basket of services covered and the patient population targeted are essential features. Bundled payments can draw on historical cost data to inform the tariff. Increasingly, bundled payments are being linked to quality requirements which must be met to receive the full payment. Bundled payments also tend to introduce an additional degree of financial risk for providers, as they may end up providing more services than the bundle has allowed for.

Table 3.1 Predominant criteria for setting bundled payments

	Episode-based bundled payments	Bundled payments for patients with a chronic condition
Range of services covered (bundled payments cover a set of services possibly across more than one setting)	Inpatient activities (e.g. elective surgery), pre and post intervention visits for a set period of time	Care related to the chronic condition such as check-ups, specialist appointments, diagnostic tests
Patient population	A certain level of poor functionality tends to be required to receive the intervention such as patients needing surgery (excluding high-risk patients)	Patient with the relevant condition
Setting the bundled payment tariff	Typically a defined budget to cover a set of services that might draw on historical costs. Recently some countries may use clinical guidelines to define "best practice" and inform tariff setting. Tariff may incorporate a "warranty" component.	A defined budget to cover a set of services that might draw on historical costs and/or best practice as defined in clinical guidelines
Financial risk	Providers bear risk to provide more services than what is covered for some patients. In addition providers might be exposed to some financial penalties if the budget is reduced when they do not meet specific criteria (e.g. quality targets)	Providers bear risk to provide more services than what is covered for some patients. In addition providers might be exposed to some financial penalties if the budget is reduced when they do not meet specific criteria (e.g. quality targets)
Financial rewards	Some forms of bundled payments include rewards for co-operation between providers or for meeting certain quality targets such as patient reported outcome measures	Some forms of bundled payments include rewards for cooperation between providers or for meeting certain quality targets such as reporting on certain intermediate or process indicators (e.g. reporting and registering HbA1c levels for diabetes)

Source: Authors' compilation.

Bundled payments aim to address all or some of the following policy objectives: improving co-ordination, quality; or productive efficiency. While DRG-type bundled payments incentivise technical efficiency, they can undermine quality. They expose purchasers to the financial risk of expensive follow-up care uncovered by the DRG payment in case of low quality treatment. More recently, the extension of bundled payments to pre- and post-patient care and the inclusion of evidence guideline-based pricing are responses to these concerns. Some countries have taken this one step further and are at various stages of developing payments partly conditioned on outcome measures to assure high quality care.

Bundled payment initiatives in the United States

While early initiatives on bundled payments in the United States began about 25 years ago, this section presents some recent efforts arising from the public and private sector.

ProvenCare bundled payment

In the private sector, the Geisinger Health System, a large integrated health care delivery system located in Central and North-Eastern Pennsylvania implemented a bundled payment system called ProvenCare in 2006 for coronary artery bypass graft surgery (CABG) (Casale et al., 2007; Paulus et al., 2008). While the aim was part of Geisinger's broader approach that emphasised quality improvement programmes, this initiative also aimed to test whether an evidence-based approach could be implemented successfully. All three hospitals part of the Geisinger Health System participated and lasted from 2006 to 2007.

The payment included services related to pre-operative care, hospital surgery, and post-discharge care (e.g. follow-up care, smoking cessation counselling, cardiac rehabilitation). This included rehospitalisations related to post-operative complications within 90 days of surgery.

The Geisinger Health System offered a bundled payment to the participating hospitals. The bundled payment also included an allowance referred to as a "warranty." This warranty was calculated using historical data and was set at 50% of the mean cost of post-operative readmissions.

The ProvenCare programme intended to reengineer its care processes to better reflect the recent changes to CABG guidelines that the American Heart Association had recently updated. Twenty guidelines were adopted and translated into 40 elements of care. These changes established standardised protocols of care.

Successful adherence to ProvenCare processes was included as one component of the surgeon's individual compensation, but not clinical outcomes to minimise any reluctance to care for high-risk patients (Casale et al., 2007). Geisinger has since added the following diagnoses to ProvenCare: elective coronary angioplasty (PCI); bariatric surgery for obesity; perinatal care; and treatment for chronic conditions (Lee et al. 2012; Delbanco, 2014).

PROMETHEUS bundled payment

In 2008, the PROMETHEUS (Provider Payment Reform for Outcomes, Margins, Evidence, Transparency, Hassle Reduction, Excellence, Understandability, and Sustainability) bundled payment model was designed to cover either an episode of care or services for a patient with a chronic condition for 21 defined clinical episodes, including for instance hip replacement and diabetes (Hussey et al., 2011). PROMETHEUS was managed and implemented by the Health Care Incentives Improvement Institute, a non-profit organisation. Payers, including health plans and self-insured employers, and health care delivery organisations at three sites volunteered to participate in the pilot and its evaluation (Hussey et al., 2011).

The general aim was to decrease health care spending while improving quality by creating a financial incentive for providers to eliminate services that were clinically ineffective or duplicative (Hussey et al., 2011). The bundled payment model was considered a "road test" to assess the effectiveness of bundled payments.

The bundled payment model intended to cover all the care required to treat a defined clinical episode. Services recommended by clinical guidelines or experts were used to inform the bundled payment, referred to as "evidence-informed case rates". The model provided the pilot sites a methodology to help set the bundled payment amount using information on historical cost and utilisation patterns, including avoidable complications. The methodology sought to ensure that the costs of avoidable complications would not be greater than the bundled payment and also intended to help providers and payers negotiate rates.

Acute care episodes Medicare demonstration

A 2009 bundled payment Medicare demonstration focussed on acute care episodes (ACE) for 37 inpatient cardiac and orthopaedic procedures. The demonstration intended to improve the quality of care, increase collaboration among providers, and reduce Medicare payments for acute care services by using market mechanisms (IMPAQ International, 2013). Five hospital sites participated. The demonstration period lasted from 2009 to 2012.

The bundled payment covered the Part A and Part B services[1] provided to Medicare FFS beneficiaries during an inpatient stay for cardiac valve and other major cardiothoracic valve, cardiac defibrillator implant, CABG, cardiac pacemaker implant or revision, percutaneous coronary intervention, and hip or knee replacement or revision (IMPAQ International, 2013).

Each site could negotiate its own discounts from Medicare. For example, one hospital site absorbed a discount of 8.25% while its physicians received full Medicare payments; in another site, both the hospital and physicians accepted discounts of 4.4% (Calsyn et al., 2014). The ACE demonstration centered on: enhanced co-ordination of care, cost-control incentives, adoption of standardised clinical protocols, and quality improvement activities (IMPAQ International, 2013). In addition, the demonstration introduced two other features that differed from the 1991 Medicare demonstration (Nelson, 2012): first it allowed for shared savings with patients where CMS shared up to 50% of the Medicare savings in the form of payments (up to a certain limit) to offset patients' Medicare cost-sharing obligations. Second, gainsharing was allowed between hospitals and doctors; they were eligible to receive a share of the savings for implementing improvements in efficiency and quality (IMPAQ International, 2013).

Integrated Healthcare Association (IHA) demonstration

In 2010, the Integrated Healthcare Association (IHA) participated in a bundled payment demonstration in California for orthopaedic surgery. The demonstration aimed to test whether bundled payment was an effective method of payment for orthopaedic surgery for commercially insured Californians younger than age 65 (Ridgely et al., 2014). A three-year grant of USD 2.9 million from the Agency for Healthcare Research and Quality provided the funding to test and evaluate the demonstration. Initially, six of California's largest health plans, eight hospitals, and an independent practice association planned to participate for the three-year duration of the demonstration.

Two episodes of care were defined: total knee replacement and total hip replacement. The services were to include facility, professional and medical implant device charges for the inpatient stay; a 90-day post-surgical warranty for related complications and readmissions. Prices were to be negotiated between the health plans and the hospitals.

Payment reform in England

Best Practice Tariffs in hospitals

A 2008 review of the National Health Service (NHS) in England found a substantial amount of non-compliance with best practice for hospital services (Darzi, 2008). As a result, a policy commitment was made to set some tariffs that financially incentivise providers to provide care compliant with best practice – referred to as Best Practice Tariffs (BPTs). The aim of this approach was to encourage the payment of services that followed clinical guidelines and to discourage variation in practice that did not follow best practice. This method of pricing was an extension to the existing system of pricing in England referred to as Healthcare Resource Group (HRG) that reflected average cost.

BPTs have different objectives, such as changing the setting of care (e.g. inpatient to day-case or day-case to outpatient setting), streamlining the pathway of care or increasing the provision of high-quality care based on best available evidence (Van de Voorde et al., 2013). The reform to the payment system is intended to encourage care that is evidence-based, focus on day cases, and reduce the number of outpatient appointments following surgery (Gershlick, 2016a).

The BPTs target hospital activities according to the following criteria: high potential impact (e.g. volume, significant unexplained variation in practice, or significant impact of best practice on outcomes); strong evidence on best practice and clinical consensus on characteristics of best practice (Van de Voorde et al., 2013). In 2010, BPTs applied to all providers of NHS-funded care, including both NHS and independent providers, for hospital admissions related to: hip fracture, stroke, cholecystectomy, and cataract surgery.

The BPTs can be higher or lower than HRG tariffs based on national average costs. The price differential between best practice and usual care is calculated to ensure that the anticipated costs of undertaking best practice are reimbursed, while creating an incentive for providers to shift from usual care to best practice. For example, the BPT for stroke is designed as a base tariff paid for all stroke patients irrespective of performance, and extra performance payments are paid out for a) rapid brain imaging, b) treating the patient in an acute stroke unit, and c) alteplase.

Coverage of BPT has steadily increased from four in 2010 to more than 50 procedures. The tariffs are set centrally and until 2016/17 were under the authority of Monitor (the pricing authority of the NHS) and now under the authority of NHS Improvement, which leaves very little room in principle for local price negotiation between providers and commissioners although there are some non-mandatory BPTs.

Bundled payment for maternity care

A completely new bundled approach was established to pay for maternity care. The maternity pathway payment approach was introduced to address two main issues arising from the previous episode-based payment system in England (Department of Health, 2016). First, organisations were paid for each inpatient admission, hospital visit, ultrasound scan, caesarean sections so the more clinical interventions were performed, the more a hospital received. The financial incentive to do more clinical interventions likely led to unnecessary care that was not appropriate and encouraged overuse. Furthermore, this may have been counter to some patients' interests who benefit most from fewer clinical interventions, closer to home. Second, NHS organisations described and recorded ante-natal and post-natal non-delivery activities in different ways, despite changes implemented every year to attempt to resolve these problems. The new payment system brought together types of care that were previously funded in different ways: FFS for certain activities such as scans, hospital visits, episode-based tariffs which were used for inpatient care (e.g. natural delivery, caesarean section) while community ante-natal and post-natal care and some other elements were funded through block contracts, designed locally that were not covered by mandatory national prices.

The objective of the new system was to allocate resources more efficiently while keeping the budget constant. The policy aim was to encourage efficient outcome-focussed care. The total level of payment was therefore set on the basis of the total reported costs of current maternity care for the three stages, ante-natal, delivery and post-natal care. For payment purposes, the pathway was split into three stages: ante-natal, delivery and post-natal care per women, with supplementary payments for specific complications. Payments were adjusted for medical needs but did not depend on delivery method (caesarean or vaginal birth).

Women choose their lead provider for each stage of the pathway. Clinical Commissioning Groups are responsible for purchasing the care and pay once for each of the three stages. This could mean three separate payments to the same lead provider or three payments to different lead providers. Where a woman chooses or is referred to another provider for an element of their care, the second provider invoices the first provider. Published business rules provide transparent instructions on what to do if a woman changes residential address and therefore commissioner during their pregnancy.

A maternity minimum dataset was established to collect information related to the new payment system. The policy applied to all organisation and was first trialled (shadow year) in 2012 and then mandated in the national tariffs in 2013 but no assessment has yet been published (Department of Health, 2016).

Moving to a value-based system in Sweden

Sweden has introduced bundled payments to replace existing payment systems. This was first initiated in Stockholm county in 2009 to respond to specific concerns regarding waiting times and the lack of quality control for hip and knee surgery. The overall health system policy focus shifted towards patient centeredness to ensure the best possible health for the population, based on available resources and more attractive work environments for health professionals in Sweden.

A working group was established with representatives of the county's public and private orthopaedic providers. These discussions led to an agreement to create a bundled payment for hip and knee surgery. All major hospitals (6), of which one was private and three private specialised centres, participated.

The bundle (referred to as OrthoChoice) included a pre-operative visit, the operation itself (including the prosthesis), inpatient care, all physician fees, and related costs (e.g. personnel costs, drugs, tests, imaging), and a follow-up visit within two years (Porter et al., 2014a). The bundle included an expected inpatient stay of six days including physical therapy and included a warranty that held providers financially liable for complications related to the surgery, such as infection or need for revision or reoperation for up to five years. For any complication a provider believed was not related to the operation or post-operative care, he/she could request an impartial expert review. Explicit criteria were used to select a homogenous group of patients with specific clinical conditions, excluding complicated patients. The bundle was not adjusted for shorter or longer hospitalisations and outpatient rehabilitation was not included.

Historical cost data and the national register data on the cost of addressing complications were used to inform the bundle payment rate. This was not a straightforward task as the cost data reported by provider varied by as much as two-fold across counties. A unique price was finally set at SEK 56 300 (USD 8 728). Payments to private providers were 6% higher to cover VAT, yielding SEK 59 678 (Porter et al., 2014a). Providers were required to maintain a reporting rate of 98% to the national quality register to receive the full payment. The national quality registers in Sweden collect individual patient data on medical diagnoses, interventions performed, and some outcomes (Porter et al., 2014a). Delivery of care changed including benchmarking and standardising care, new manuals and checklists; the mandatory accreditation of providers by county, and extra post-operative visits to help with recovery.

Following the pilot for hip and knee replacement, a new pilot for spine surgery was launched in 2013 developed in collaboration with the Stockholm County Council, the Swedish Society of Spinal Surgeons and the Ivbar Institute.

In 2013, Sweden established a nationwide collaboration (SVEUS). This collaboration aimed to establish a new analysis platform for Swedish health care to support continuous clinical improvement, research and steering including reimbursement. The focus was to enable monitoring of value (case-mix adjusted outcomes and cost). The stakeholders include the Ministry of Health and Social Affairs, Ivbar Institute, county councils, the Karolinska Institute, and health professionals. The Ministry of Health and Social Affairs, together with the counties, funded the five-year pilot that began in 2013 (EUR 8 million) in eight priority areas: spine surgery, osteoarthritis, obstetric care, bariatric surgery, stroke, diabetes, osteoporosis, and breast cancer. The monitoring platform was set up by the participating counties jointly but payment systems were implemented separately by each county council/region, according to their requirements. Projects are scheduled for completion in 2017.

3.3. Payments are used to improve the quality of care for chronic conditions

A number of countries have established evidence-based guidelines and comprehensive care strategies to enhance health outcomes for chronic patients by overcoming care fragmentation in the delivery of care. For example, the Netherlands started to experiment with bundled payments for common chronic diseases such as diabetes, cardiovascular diseases and COPD in 2007. Taking this a step further, innovative payment models target high-cost chronic conditions for which a smaller number of patients are affected as seen in Portugal and the Netherlands.

Bundled payments for chronic conditions in Portugal

In Portugal, hospital outpatient services were reimbursed by FFS for medical consultations and for day-centre episodes without considering patient diagnosis (demand side) or resource consumption (supply side). This system placed upward pressure on volume of services, encouraged overprovision of medical consultations and day centre appointments (which yielded a higher tariff than medical consultations). Hospitals treating a large number of patients diagnosed with high-cost chronic conditions incurred financial losses. This possibly led to cherry-picking strategies and suboptimal quality of care. There were also potentially difficulties in accessing state-of-the art health care (e.g. innovative treatments), and few hospitals were offering comprehensive care for chronic conditions such as cancer, forcing patients to visit different hospitals or hospital settings to access care. Additionally, statistical data were scarce and data on quality of care were anecdotal (Lourenço, 2016).

To address these problems, and shift policy focus towards more patient-oriented care and comprehensive disease management programmes, the Portuguese National Health Service introduced a bundled payment for patients with selected chronic conditions beginning in 2007. Tariffs were set to follow clinical guidelines for high-cost conditions that require medical consultations and other outpatient services (e.g. hospital day care, hospital drug costs, diagnostic and therapeutic exams).

A one-year pilot was run first for patients with HIV/AIDS. The payment model was first applied to hospitals with more than 400 patients and then extended to all hospitals treating HIV/AIDS patients. The bundled payment covered all outpatient treatment provided to HIV/AIDS patients who had not yet been treated with antiretroviral therapy, including, ancillary diagnostic and therapeutic exams.

The bundled tariff was determined according to clinical guidelines for patient follow up, including a number of medical appointments, diagnostic exams, and therapeutic regimen. The list of services included was endorsed by patient associations and medical doctor representatives.

The payment consisted of a monthly tariff per capita to cover all services. To receive the payment, hospitals were required to: 1) provide required reporting (e.g. report on the percentage of patients that comply with treatment; percentage of patients with controlled infection levels); 2) report on undetectable viral load after 24 weeks of treatment; 3) provide at least two medical appointments, two viral loads and two contacts with the pharmacist per year. If the costs were below the bundled payment, hospitals kept the savings. If the costs were above the payment, the hospitals were responsible for covering the financial loss. A specific Electronic Health Record was developed to support patient treatment and additional funding was provided for implementation and set up costs in hospitals. Since 2009, the payment model was extended to all hospitals and in 2012 it was extended to all patients with HIV/AIDS including those already on antiretroviral drugs. The tariff was adjusted to reflect the average costs incurred by hospitals.

Following a positive assessment of this initiative, the government used the following criteria to extend the initiative to other high-cost conditions: a) high ambulatory treatment cost; b) existence of clinical guidelines and clinical pathways; c) availability of data to enable costing and pricing. The high-cost conditions include multiple sclerosis, pulmonary hypertension, lysosomal storage diseases, familial amyloid polyneuropathy and selected oncological diseases (i.e. breast cancer, cervix cancer, colon-rectal cancer). For example in the case of oncology diseases, the payment model emphasises patient-centered care and includes all care during 24 months (inpatient such as surgery) and different outpatient services (radiotherapy, chemotherapy, ancillary exams). These high-cost conditions are under evaluation by the Ministry of Health and independent groups but results are not yet available. In 2014, close to 10% of the overall hospital funding from the central government was channelled through this new payment model (Lourenço, 2016).

Bundled payment in the Netherlands

Diabetes bundled payments

In 2007, the Netherlands implemented bundled payments for select chronic conditions (type 2 diabetes, COPD and cardiovascular disease risk management) with the aim of improving the delivery of care for patients with chronic conditions.

The bundled payment for type 2 diabetic patients defines a single payment per patient for all standard diabetic care. Participation of providers and payers is voluntary. The bundled payment is made to care groups. These care groups are legal entities established as part of the reform, largely comprised of GPs. Care groups either provide the required care services themselves or in most cases sub-contract to health professionals to deliver them. The service elements included in the bundled payment have been defined on a national level by the National Diabetes Foundation and were agreed between associations of providers and patients and refer to primary care only. They are fully covered by mandatory insurance without additional payments for patients. In general, the contract between insurer and care groups contains the same service components. There are few differences between services recommended by the National Diabetes Foundation and those included in the bundled payment activities for the ten analysed care groups, mainly referring to services which are not precisely defined in the national standards (Table 3.2) (Struijs et al., 2012a).

Table 3.2. Diabetes bundled payment in sample of care groups compared with National Diabetes Foundation recommendations, the Netherlands

	NDF care standard	Provided by care groups
Diagnostic phase		
Formal diagnosis	No	None
Initial risk assessment	Yes	All
Treatment and standard check-ups		
12-month check-ups	Yes	All
3-month check-ups	Yes	All
Obtaining fundus images	Yes	All
Evaluating fundus images	Yes	All
Foot examinations	Yes	All
Supplementary foot exams	Unclear	All
Foot care	No	None
Laboratory testing	Yes	Most
Smoking cessation support	Yes	None
Exercise counselling	Yes	All
Supervised exercising	No	None
Dietary counselling	Yes	All
Prescribing medicines	No	Some
Insulin initiation	No	All
Insulin adjustment	No	All
Psychosocial care	No	None
Medical aids	No	None
Additional GP consultations (diabetes-related)	Unclear	All
Additional GP consultations (non-related)	No	None
Specialist advice	Yes	All

Source: Adapted from Struijs et al. (2012a).

Tariffs and activities were negotiated between health insurers and care groups. In the case that care groups sub-contract other health professionals, the price for treatment was negotiated between the care group and the individual provider (Figure 3.1). The method of payment for services provided by sub-contractors was also negotiable with care groups – such as FFS, a fixed rate, or salary.

Figure 3.1. Schematic approaches to bundled payment in the Netherlands

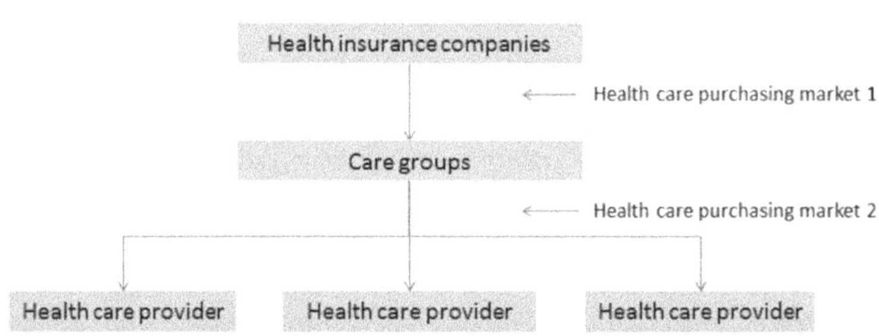

Source: Struijs et al. (2012a).

Without waiting for the findings of an evaluation of this approach, the Dutch Parliament voted in September 2009 to institutionalise the process for both type 2 diabetes and cardiovascular risk management, starting in January 2010, and for COPD, starting in July 2010 (Struijs et al., 2010). In 2010, there were 100 care groups in the Netherlands consisting of an average of 46 general practitioners who delivered care to an average of 3 149 diabetes patients each with about 19 insurers having contracts per care group (Struijs et al., 2012b).

Tackling Parkinson's disease through delivery reform

Care for patients with Parkinson's disease was characterised by high costs, sub-optimal care and dissatisfied patients. Being a relatively rare disease, provider expertise to treat this condition was low, and there were little incentives – or means – for the individual provider to improve delivery of care (Vlaanderen et al., 2016). In 2004, ParkinsonNet (PN), an academic non-profit initiative led by Radboud University Medical Centre (UMC) and the Dutch association of neurologists was piloted as a regional network. The aim was first to deliver patient-centered care more efficiently without any changes to how providers were paid.

The programme was later expanded to cover the entire country via regional networks composed of a multidisciplinary group of 19 types of health professionals (geriatricians, neurologists, occupational therapist, etc.), for treatment in primary, secondary and tertiary care. Providers have to meet certain quality standards to join a regional network including treating a minimum number of patients. The providers work more closely according to the scientific guidelines. The ParkinsonNet Coordination & Innovation Centre (C&I centre) oversees training and ensuring appropriate distribution of providers and a regional co-ordinator manages the local network (Vlaanderen et al., 2016).

Patients can visit PN and non-PN providers. However, some insurance companies recently decided to contract only PN members for the care for Parkinson's disease, creating financial disincentives for patients visiting non-PN providers. The Dutch association of health insurance companies (Zorgverzekeraars Nederland, ZN) financed 50% of ParkinsonNet with providers' membership fees financing the rest. The annual costs to maintain and co-ordinate the network of ParkinsonNet are EUR 1.5 million.

The next phase is to introduce a bundled payment to further improve the delivery of care. In the new payment model, insurers will pay a population-based budget to the PN networks. The budget will be based on the expected Parkinson's disease-related health care cost of the insured population for both primary and secondary care. A shared savings model will be permitted in which the savings will be divided between insurers and providers with no restriction on how the providers spend these savings. A portion of the payment will be linked to health care outcomes.

Further details of the payment model have yet to be finalised. It is not yet known how the budget exactly will be calculated, and how it will be managed, or when the outcome-based payments will be incorporated. Second, it is also not clear how the regional networks will divide the budgets between the professions and the individual providers, who will be responsible when the budgets are exceeded, and how the financial consequences will be divided between insurers and providers (Vlaanderen et al., 2016).

Bundled payment for diabetes in Denmark

In Denmark, the government introduced a new bundled payment policy in 2007 that targeted diabetes. The aim of the policy was to ensure the quality of diabetic care provided in general practice with a shift towards more integrated care where GPs could play a pivotal role in care co-ordination (Rudkjøbing et al., 2015). General practitioners could voluntarily choose to participate in the new payment policy.

The bundled payment included an annual consultation and the co-ordination of specialist services such as eye care, endocrinology, and podiatry. To receive the payment, GPs were required to report key data from the electronic health record system, which generated reports for each practice, based on quality indicators (Rudkjøbing et al., 2015). They were also required to use a specific IT system and would be entitled to a related one-off payment of approximately EUR 1 000 to use it. The bundled tariff rate was negotiated between representatives from stakeholder groups in the regions and the municipalities and the Ministry of Finance. The annual tariff was set at EUR 156 for each diabetic patient following an annual extensive consultation with the GP. This payment would replace the existing capitation and FFS payment of EUR 17 per consultation for GPs who opted to participate in the new payment policy. The new payment policy was based on redistribution under the negotiated fixed financial level of activity for the whole population of GPs, so there was no "new" money but rather funding was shifted from other areas (Rudkjøbing et al., 2015).

Crossing health and social care boundaries for patients with long-term care needs in the United Kingdom (England)

In 2012, a pilot programme that covered the costs of health and social care relating to a person's long-term care (LTC) needs in a 12-month period was launched (Gershlick, 2016b). The aim was to deliver integrated health and social care for people who need support from multiple providers based on need rather than diagnosis. NHS England believes the model has the potential to change the payment system for up to 20 or 25% of the total health and social care budget in England. The policy focus was to shift some accountability to providers through risk sharing agreements between those who provide and those who purchase the care (Gershlick, 2016b).

The services cover primary care, acute care, and community care. This required aligning the funding flows and incentives with people's needs, rather than paying just for episodes of care. The pilot programme started in 2012 with seven early implementers. The bundled payment will be annually risk adjusted based on need. The programme has developed provisional estimate of local per-patient tariffs. "Shadow testing" was expected in 2014/15, with full implementation in 2015/16.

3.4. Key characteristics of payment reforms towards bundled payments

A summary of the information just presented according to key characteristics is found in Table 3.3 for the Netherlands, Portugal, Sweden, United Kingdom (England), and United States which highlights some of the main differences across programmes. For example, some bundled payment covers episodes of care such as hip replacement or common chronic conditions (e.g. diabetes) while others focus on high cost less prevalent conditions such as HIV/AIDS (Portugal) or Parkinson's disease (the Netherlands). Bundled payment is used in some countries for both episodes-of-care and chronic conditions (e.g. Sweden, England, United States). The basket of services provided may cover more than one setting such as primary care, and secondary care or focus on one setting. An assessment of these policy reforms is presented in the next section.

Table 3.3. Key characteristics of payment reform in selected OECD countries

	United States	United States	England	England	England	Sweden	Portugal	Netherlands	Netherlands
Type and name of payment reform	Bundled payment for acute care episodes cardiac and orthopedic care (ACE)	Bundled payment for a select number of activities and conditions (PROMETHEUS)	Best practice tariffs in hospitals (BPT)	Maternity care pathway	Bundled payment for patients with long-term care needs (Year of Care)	Bundled payment for an episode of care (SVEUS)	Bundled payment for select chronic conditions	Bundled payment for Parkinson's Disease (ParkinsonNet)	Bundled payment for diabetes, vascular risk management, COPD)
Basket of services	37 inpatient cardiac and orthopaedic procedures	Select activities that can cover primary and secondary care	50 clinical areas of hospital activities (e.g. stroke, hip fracture, cataract surgery)	Ante-natal, delivery and post-natal care	Primary care, acute care and community care	Spine surgery and follow-up care for two years	Outpatient treatment, diagnostic, therapeutic exams	Primary care, secondary care, tertiary care	Primary care and select specialist care
Patient population (conditions/episode)	Patients requiring an inpatient stay for select cardiac or orthopaedic procedures	Patients with a select episode of care (e.g. hip replacement) or a chronic condition (e.g diabetes)	Patients requiring select hospital services (e.g. stroke, hip fracture, cataract surgery)	Pregnant women	Patients requiring long-term care needs	Patients requiring spine surgery	HIV/AIDS and other select high-cost chronic rare conditons	Parkinson's disease	Type 2 diabetic patients, vascular risk management and COPD
Providers involved	Hospitals and physicians belonging to a facility in each participating site	Three pilot sites where two focussed on chronic conditions and the third focussed on procedures	Public hospitals	Public hospitals and midwifery teams, and birth centres	Multiple providers that offer health and social care services	Public hospitals	Public hospitals	17 types of health professionals	Care groups of providers typically managed by GPs that include other health professionals (e.g. nurses)

Source: Authors' compilation.

3.5. Assessment of payment reforms

This section assesses the payment reforms in select countries according to two main criteria: whether intended policy objectives were met (such as achieving quality gains and/or savings) and the conditions for implementation that either encouraged or hindered implementation.

In a number of cases, cost savings were made, and typically when quality of care (e.g. reduced readmission rates, patient satisfaction) was measured no deterioration was observable across available indicators of quality. In other cases some improvements in quality occurred following the payment reform, although sometimes at a higher cost (Table 3.4). While bundled payments show quality improvements, and generate savings, the gains depend on the condition or episode targeted. Typically, the introduction of bundled payment was part of a larger reform. Stakeholder support led to improved protocols of care, pilots were successful. Tariffs tend to draw on historical costs, sometimes with normative adjustments aiming to reflect clinical guidelines or adjustments to incorporate treatment outcome information. However there are challenges including tariff setting can be complex, bundled payments shift some financial risk onto the provider, and increase the administrative burden.

Table 3.4. Assessment of bundle payment reform in select OECD countries

	United States	United States	England	England	England	Sweden	Portugal	Netherlands	Netherlands
Type and name of payment reform	Bundled payment for acute care episodes cardiac and orthopedic care (ACE)	Bundled payment for a select number of chronic conditions (PROMETHEUS)	Best practice tariffs in hospitals (BPT)	Maternity care pathway	Bundled payment for patients with long-term care needs	Bundled payment for an episode of care (SVEUS)	Bundled payment for select chronic conditions	Bundled payment for Parkinson's disease (ParkinsonNet)	Bundled payment for diabetes (select chronic conditions)
Assessment of policy impact									
Achievement in terms of policy objective :									
Quality	+	Various issues delayed implementation	+/-	Evaluation not yet available	Evaluation not yet available	+	+	+ (Before payment reform)	+
Savings	+	Various issues delayed implementation		Reduction in caesarean section rate but savings evaluation not yet available	Evaluation not yet available	+	+	+ (Before payment reform)	-
Unintended consequences		Various issues delayed implementation						Competition concern	
Conditions for implementation									
Payment reform embedded in larger policy reform	+	+	+	+	+	+	+	-	+
Stakeholder participation in policy development (e.g. actively consulted in establishment of law/scheme)	+	+	+	+	+	+	+	+	+
Payer participation	Mandatory	Mandatory	Mandatory	Mandatory	Mandatory	Mandatory	Mandatory	Voluntary	Voluntary
Provider participation	Voluntary	Voluntary	Mandatory	Mandatory	Mandatory	Voluntary	Voluntary	Voluntary	Voluntary
Administrative burden		+	+	+	Not yet known			+	+
Data collection and use	New and existing data	New and existing data	Existing data	New and existing data	New and existing data	Existing data	EHR established	New and existing data	New and existing data
How are tariffs set?	Bundle of Medicare Part A and Medicare Part B services and negotiated at each site	PROMETHEUS developed a platform to assist in setting tariffs using evidenced-based rates	Tariff reflects best practice extends current system of average costs	Total costs of antenatal, delivery and postnatal care	Annually risk-adjusted capitated funding model based on need.	Tariffs set to reflect clinical guidelines and can include follow-up, warranty payment and outcome information	According to clinical guidelines such as follow up, number of medical appointments, diagnostic exams, and therapeutic regimen	Capitated payment currently being piloted	Negotiated between care groups and insurers while subcontractors negotiate their own payments
Independent evaluation of reform	+	+	+			+	+	+	+

Source: Authors' compilation.

Achieving policy objectives

In a number of cases, initiatives for bundled payments for acute care episodes and chronic conditions saw improvements in the quality of care, while for other experimentations quality levels were maintained at a lower cost of provision. The deterioration of quality was also reported in one instance. Most initiatives in acute care succeeded in reducing costs per treatment. The potential to generate savings appears less clear for bundled payments than for chronic conditions. In the Netherlands, bundled payments for diabetes patients led to cost increases.

The three-year ACE demonstration saved Medicare USD 319 per episode of care for a total of approximately USD 4 million in net savings for 12 501 episodes of care. But one negative quality result was reported: there was a reduction in the use of internal mammary artery grafts in patients undergoing coronary artery bypass graft (CABG) surgery because there was an incentive to reduce cost (operating room time). Surgeons may have moved away from a technically more complex approach, but one that has been shown to improve outcomes (IMPAQ International, 2013). The short duration of the demonstration, however, may have made it difficult to observe quality improvements (IMPAQ International, 2013). Apart from that, other detrimental impacts on quality were not observed: sicker patients were not excluded, nor were there increased transfers to post-acute facilities. The proposed financial incentives for patients (shared savings) did not appear to influence patient choice of hospital which remained driven by reputation or referral by their primary care physician. Stakeholders suggested extending incentives to primary care physicians or referring physicians— who directly influence where a beneficiary receives health care (IMPAQ International, 2013; Calsyn et al., 2014).

The Geisinger ProvenCare bundled payment for CABG, showed positive results. A study using clinical outcome data on consecutive elective CABG patients seen in the 12 months pre-intervention were compared with a post-intervention group (Berry et al., 2009). Initially, 59% of patients received the required standards of care and by the end of the study, compliance reached 100%. Clinical outcomes showed improved trends in eight out of nine measured areas (e.g., patient readmissions to intensive care units decreased from 2.9% to 0.9% and blood products usage decreased from 23.4% to 16.2%). Operative mortality decreased to zero. ProvenCare also achieved a 10% reduction in readmissions, shorter average length of stay, and reduced hospital charges.

BPTs in England, which were an extension to existing HRGs, show good results for certain conditions but less clear for others. For hip fractures, for example, patients treated under the BPT were more likely to receive surgery within 48 hours after admission which was a condition of payment and a lower mortality rate was recorded for them (Marshal et al., 2014). On the other hand, no beneficial impact of the stroke BPT on national quality and outcome indicators was found but this was partly due to improvements already achieved nationally through additional activities to improve the quality of stroke care (McDonald et al., 2012).

With regards to the payment for maternity care in England, recent data show that compared with Scotland which did not introduce the bundled payment, there has been a levelled trend in caesarean sections suggesting a possible reduction in the overprovision of caesarean sections (Figure 3.2) (Department of Health, 2016).

Figure 3.2. Elective caesarean births in England and Scotland before and after April 2013, United Kingdom

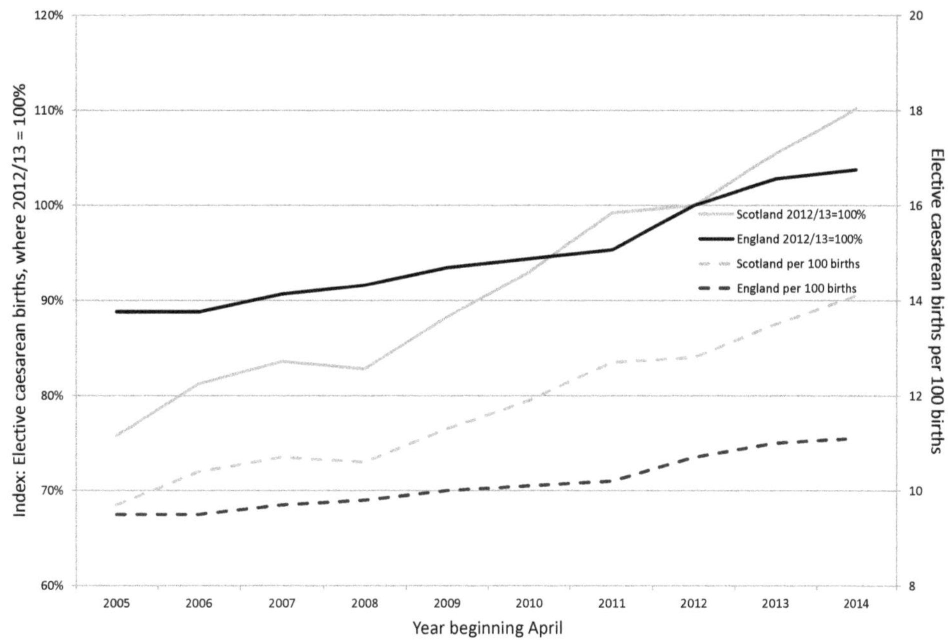

Source: Health and Social Care Information Centre, Scottish Morbidity Record 02 (SMR02), ISD Scotland.

In Sweden, the Stockholm pilot for hip and knee surgery showed a reduction in waiting times, costs (20%) and complications (26%) (Porter et al., 2014b). The recent pilot of spine surgery also showed reductions in average length of stay and cost per patient, as well as a reduction in complications from surgery (Wohlin et al., 2016).

In Portugal, the first set of results of the implementation of a bundled payment showed that the average cost for treating HIV/AIDS patients decreased while the quality of care was maintained as measured by patient adherence to medication, controlled infection levels, and compliance of providers with the treatment guidelines (Lourenço, 2016).

In the Netherlands, the bundled payment for diabetes showed improvements in quality but costs increased. An evaluation showed that most process indicators showed improvements (HbA1c, BMI checked and blood pressure checked; improvements in kidney function and cholesterol tests) (Struijs et al., 2012a). The number of annual eye tests declined due to changes in contracts to biannual tests. Most of the patient outcome measures showed modest improvement (meeting blood pressure and cholesterol targets), but HbA1c level rose slightly due to longer diabetes duration and no change in BMI. Composite process indicators showed improvement but not consistently across all care groups (Struijs et al., 2012a). Despite a reduction in the use of specialist care (25%), costs increased by EUR 288 for diabetes patients enrolled in the bundled payment scheme. The reasons are unclear and may be due to delaying the use of specialist care which could have resulted in more costly care, or the most expensive procedures (Hasaart, 2011). There is no evidence that diabetic patients with and without co-morbidities received different levels of care (de Bruin et al., 2013). Patients were satisfied with their care but were not necessarily aware that they were part of the scheme for diabetes care (Struijs et al., 2012b).

Unintended consequences

Diverging interests and financial risk impede implementation

Some initiatives encountered problems with implementation. In the IHA Bundled Episode Payment and Gainsharing Demonstration in California for orthopaedic surgery, an agreement was difficult to reach on bundle definitions. Payers were interested in defining large bundles while providers wanted to define narrow ones focussed on low-risk patients. Health plans wanted to negotiate lower prices and to set payments that would be less than FFS while hospitals wanted a higher level payment than under FFS and were concerned about taking on financial risk. In the end, the definition of the bundled payment was narrow (e.g. excluded obese patients, post-acute and rehabilitation services), which did not make it economically viable. Exposure to financial risk resulted in a couple of the largest payers exiting the demonstration before it began. With no mechanism to attract patients (e.g. lower out-of-pocket payments to participate) hospitals were less keen to participate. The low level of participation raised problems to implement the payment scheme: there were only 35 surgeries carried out in the health plans and 111 in ambulatory surgery centers, which made evaluation impossible (Ridgely et al., 2014).

Similarly, the PROMETHEUS bundled payment model initiated in 2008 has not been implemented so far for lack of agreement on the setting of prices and in particular accounting for potentially avoidable complications and the sharing of the related financial risk (Hussey et al., 2011).

In Denmark, the bundled payment policy for diabetic care had a slow start after its introduction in 2007. Participation among GPs varied in the five Danish regions with an average of 30% by 2012, ranging from around 20% in the Central Region to 40% in the Capital Region (Rudkjøbing et al., 2015). While the participating practices covered about a third of the Danish patient population, only about 10% of all diabetic patients were treated in the participating practices. Take up was higher among younger physicians. Among those that joined the policy, other attractive features included a more systematic approach to treatment and opportunity for documentation and research (Thorsen, 2008). For older physicians, a barrier to take up the policy was time to retirement as it was not seen to be worthwhile to switch to the bundled payment policy (Thorsen, 2008).

The financial incentive of the bundled payment, however, contributed to the slow take up. The amount was not risk-adjusted and may have discouraged GPs to join particularly for those with a patient population that was difficult to manage. A feasibility study conducted in 2007 before the implementation of the policy suggested that for quite sick diabetic patients, the financial incentive might not be sufficient and act as a barrier for GPs to join (Thorsen, 2007). A qualitative study carried out one year after the policy was implemented found that some GPs were not incentivised by the amount of the bundled payment to join (Thorsen, 2008). The funding for the policy was a redistribution of existing resources which might have discouraged GPs to join as some perceived that participating in the new policy would mean taking away money from other GPs. In addition, the EUR 1 000 offered to GPs to implement the required IT system was not seen to be sufficient for some GPs (Thorsen, 2008). Lastly, the feasibility study revealed a worry among GPs about increased external control and monitoring of quality (Thorsen, 2007).

The low success in participation of the payment policy led the government to abandon it in 2014. However, the data capture system has been detached from the diabetes fee and has now been extended to all patient groups.

Competition concerns in the Netherlands

For Parkinson's disease, it remains to be seen whether the new payment model will be at odds with competition laws applicable to the Dutch health system: namely whether the Parkinson provider networks can be considered as monopolies limiting competition among providers in the treatment of patients with Parkinson's disease. Within the regional network, the majority of the patients would be treated by PN providers, leaving little competition between PN providers and non-PN providers (Vlaanderen et al., 2016).

3.6. Conditions for implementing payment reform

Stakeholder support necessary

The positive results of some of the bundling initiatives with regards to quality and spending control in part owe to stakeholder engagement and support. Continued support by all actors can be challenging as it may require balancing opposing interests, in particular between purchaser and provider. In the Medicare demonstration, the discounted payment rates were negotiated for the ACE demonstration but the discount varied by site. A large part of the savings came from negotiating lower prices for medical devices. Hospitals and physicians were allowed to share in savings but they had to meet quality and monitoring requirements (Calsyn et al., 2014).

There was also provider support in both England and Sweden and patients support for the changes in Sweden. In England, clinical stakeholders were involved in informing the BPTs. In Sweden, researchers from several universities in relevant disciplines such as medicine and health economics were involved to inform the pricing of services. A wide group of stakeholders were involved including health professionals, and local authorities. SVEUS's national steering group set targets, scope, organisation and budget and monitored development. The work was carried out as 12 subprojects led by a participating county council. The subgroups contained representatives from participating county councils, relevant national specialist associations, national quality registries, patient associations and Ivbar Institute.

In Portugal, the payment reform was led by the Central Administration for the Health System, involving different stakeholders according to the condition analysed (Lourenço, 2016). Wide stakeholder engagement was a catalyst for implementation. The main partner for the development of the payment reform was the Directorate General of Health, the entity responsible for issuing clinical guidelines. Clinical experts, providers and, in some cases patients associations, were also engaged in the development of the payment reform. Experts from academic institutions were invited to participate on monitoring and evaluation. However, there was some resistance among providers that were not selected as pilot or reference centres.

In the Netherlands, the move towards bundled payment for Parkinson's disease would have not been possible without strong stakeholder involvement and support. In fact, the creation of PN as a bottom-up approach was entirely driven by providers supported by patients and some health insurers. In this context, the move towards a bundled payment is the end result of restructuring of care processes and not the first step.

Improvements in protocols and standardisation of care

Bundled payment led in most countries to organisational changes in the delivery of care. Health care providers intensified their collaboration – within and across settings – and a greater standardisation of care was achieved. Generally, this was facilitated/accompanied by the development of guidelines which increased transparency in the bundled payment, the monitoring of cost and quality including feedback loops to providers.

In Sweden, the bundled payments for OrthoChoice and the payment for spine surgery in the national collaboration led to improving the process in the accreditation of providers. The professional associations played a key role to develop new manuals and checklists along with the other stakeholders (e.g. local authorities) to standardise practise and establish benchmarks (Ivbar Institute, 2015).

In the ACE demonstration in the United States, physicians and hospitals were involved in co-ordinating care and strengthened their relationship by regularly discussing methods to improve the quality of care. Hospitals provided physicians with report cards (relating to quality and their costs). Standardised protocols of care were agreed upon. Quality measures were tracked, allowing physicians and staff to more efficiently monitor and improve patient outcomes. The demonstration also encouraged hospitals and doctors to discuss and identify high quality and cost-effective devices which allowed hospitals to negotiate lower prices from medical sellers (Calsyn et al., 2014).

In the bundled payment system of ProvenCare in the United States, surgeons reviewed specific guidelines for CABG surgery and developed 19 clinically applicable recommendations. Measureable process elements were developed based on these recommendations (Berry et al., 2009). As a result, the programme established best practices for CABG patients; created a multidisciplinary team to ensure that these best practices were part of the everyday workflow; and implemented a feedback system to allow space for adapting the process of care as needed that drew on real-time reporting.

For diabetes care in the Netherlands, delivery was more structured and based on protocols. The benefit packages that insurers offered for diabetes care became more uniform across care groups over time. This was in part due to the increasing expertise among health care insurance companies and care groups. An evaluation conducted in 2010 showed that services generally included the recommended 12-month and three-month check-ups, and the annual eye and foot examinations (Struijs et al., 2010). In eight of the nine contracts studied in the 2010 evaluation, laboratory examinations, exercise and diet counselling, and specialist consultations were included. Differences in the range of services covered by individual contracts were observed for services which were not precisely defined in national standards such as foot care, and additional diabetes-related GP consultations, prescription medicines, insulin initiation and adjustment (Struijs et al., 2010; Struijs et al., 2012a).

Care standardisation is also an important element of the Parkinson networks in the Netherlands, even if they predate the introduction of the bundled payment. Members of the network are required to meet a number of minimal standards such a treating a minimum number of patients per year or the regular attendance of multi-disciplinary team meetings to discuss cases and stimulate collaboration (Vlaanderen et al., 2016).

Changing roles of health providers

In some countries the introduction of bundled payments has not only sought to incentivise better co-ordination between health care professionals within and across settings, but also resulted in a shift of tasks across providers and even changes in the scope of practice and responsibilities of selected heath care professions.

In the Netherlands, payment reform encouraged a reallocation of tasks in diabetes care. In primary care, practice nurses took on a more central role and carried most if not all the regular check-ups in GP practices, though it was reported this shift had already begun before the payment reform (Struijis et al., 2012a). More insulin-dependent patients without complications were treated in general practices. Eye examinations were conducted outside the settings of ophthalmologists such as by optometrists or general practice laboratories. There was concern among some providers that task reallocation may have a negative impact on GP practices (losing patient contact and expertise) or practice nurses may not be sufficiently trained. Practice nurses, however, devoted more time to patients and GPs had more time for other patients.

Pilot experiments proved successful

The move towards bundled payments has been frequently tested by countries for a smaller number of settings before being rolled out on a greater scale. This helped to verify whether changes in the payments system had the desired effects and allowed for adjusting incentives before general implementation.

In Portugal and the Netherlands, pilot experiments were established first which led to successful implementation nationwide. Portugal began a one-year pilot payment for HIV/AIDs in selected hospitals before expanding it nationwide two years later. In the Netherlands, evaluations of the diabetes pilot were built into the policy process when the pilot was expanded nationwide in 2009 (Struijs et al., 2010; Struijs and Baan, 2011). The bundled payment for hip and knee surgery in Sweden laid the groundwork for a national collaboration to reform payment systems there.

Before the payment reform, in the Netherlands for patients with Parkinson's disease, there was a reduction in costs for patients treated in ParkinsonNet and care improved health outcomes in terms of prevention of falls and hip fractures, reduced rehabilitation time, and reduced use of nursing homes (Beersen et al., 2011; Bloem and Munneke, 2014; Munneke et al., 2010; Nijkrake et al., 2010; Vlaanderen et al., 2016). Ultimately, the Parkinson networks aim to explore possibilities to sign outcome-based bundled payment contracts with health insurers incorporating a range of primary care and secondary care activities. As an intermediate step, a "lighter version" which uses budget allocation based on capitation for hospital care was piloted in 2014 (Vlaanderen et al., 2016). This version includes all costs for diagnostics, treatments and follow-up visits in one tariff but distinguishes between three categories of Parkinson patients based on how long they have been diagnosed with the disease.

The NHS England pilot for patients with long-term conditions is still in the early phase of implementation, but there has been development of a whole-population analysis approach which can support the development of a national funding framework, guidance on collecting the evidence required to demonstrate the effectiveness of earlier discharges from acute care, and the provision of an initial estimate of local per-patient tariffs (Gershlick, 2016b).

Bundled payments can lead to administrative burden

Moving towards bundled payment to pay health care providers can entail a certain level of additional administrative work, both for payers and providers. To set tariffs, costs for separate activities within the bundled payment need to be identified. In case the payment incorporates quality metrics, process or outcome indicators need to be measured and reported. There may be issues around exchange of information between providers if a bundled payment reflects evidence-based treatment across providers. Finally, modifications to existing billing practice may require additional guidelines if more than one provider is involved.

In England, despite provider support towards BPT payments, the changes were challenging to implement and difficult to understand for providers. The Audit Commission recommended making price setting simpler and clearer with a more transparent explanation of the BPT payment models that should be reported alongside public reporting of quality of care. Providers should also better understand the clinical guidelines attached to each BPT and commissioners should ensure completeness and accuracy of the tariff to trigger BPT payments.

Even though providers responded positively to the payment reform towards a bundled payment for maternity care in England, there was an administrative burden relating to invoicing providers for their services (Department of Health, 2016). The complexity of information did not allow for the flow of confidential data, which made it difficult for finance departments to determine the lead provider for invoicing purposes. Commissioners receive aggregated data and so were unable to identify patients correctly leaving the risk of paying twice for the same care.

For diabetes care in the Netherlands, there was poor IT integration between GP systems and care groups systems as not all providers could access the care groups system, requiring data to be entered twice into both systems. The quality of the data reporting among care group was mixed and required standardisation as health insurance companies were also not always satisfied about the quality of the accountability information they received from care groups (Struijis et al., 2012a). In a survey of providers, daily routines for shared care were still sub-optimal and facilities such as registration systems should be improved to further optimise communication and exchange of information (Raaijmakers et al., 2013).

The PROMETHEUS bundled payment developed a series of support tools for the participating pilot sites including an accounting tool that analysed insurance claims to identify services that were part of the bundle; and an analytic software that pilot sites could use to analyse their historical claims data for cost and utilisation patterns in bundles of care (Hussey et al., 2011). But the accounting tool was difficult to implement alongside existing insurance claims information and no site was able to modify its claims processing methods to identify bundled services.

In the IHA demonstration, the lack of software initially contributed to a delay in implementation. The participating health plans decided to reimburse services manually which increased administrative burden. Once software became available it was too late to test this solution as low volume hampered the pilot's viability for proper evaluation (Ridgely et al., 2014).

New data collection systems established

In some cases, the introduction of bundled payment required the collection of new data. In Portugal, new data systems had to be established, including an electronic health record. Similarly in the Netherlands, care groups in the diabetes bundled payment were increasingly using integrated information systems. All hospitals were required to collect a select number of indicators for Parkinson's disease.

The policy in Denmark led to improvements in reporting due to the required IT system that GPs had to use. Indeed quality improvements and especially the data capture systems were for some considered more important than the financial consideration when deciding on whether to join the payment policy (Thorsen, 2008).

In Sweden, embedding monitoring systems was part of the reform. Relevant monitoring measures were defined for each patient group, along with guidance on how they will be measured and monitored. The aim of the monitoring systems was to allow for rapid feedback as well as identification of anomalies and comparisons between different care providers and county councils (Ivbar Institute, 2015).

In the PROMETHEUS initiative, the pilot sites were able to improve their existing data systems and changed the way their electronic health records were used. This allowed pilot sites to rethink how to improve delivery and made them recognise data needs for measurement of quality and cost (Hussey et al., 2011).

Differing approaches to setting tariffs

The way that payments are designed and tariffs set is of vital importance for providers and payers. Different approaches have been followed by countries to set the tariffs of the bundles including identifying and pricing all services that constitute best practice along an evidence-based pathway which increases transparency and incorporating outcome measures. The extent to which bundled tariffs refer to one single payment or are made up of several payments also differs.

In England, the pricing for some models under the BPT includes a "base price" and a "BPT component", while for other models a completely new tariff was established. Although every procedure that shifts into the appropriate setting attracts a higher payment, the base payment is lower than or equal to a tariff set for the conventional way of providing care, i.e. based on the national average of reported costs across both settings (Gershlick, 2016a). Different approaches were used to set tariffs depending on the condition. The general relationship between standard or conventional tariffs, the base price and the BPT component is depicted in Figure 3.3.

For cataract surgery, establishing the value of the national tariff first involved breaking down the new, streamlined cataract pathway into existing HRG units – from initial assessment through to surgery (as a day patient) in hospital and then follow-up in the outpatient setting. The overall tariff for this new pathway was essentially the sum of the average national costs for each element of the pathway (Department of Health, 2010).

The base price or non-BPT has in some cases been reduced to become punitive, in order to incentivise use of the best practice guidelines. BPTs can be higher or lower than national average costs, and are paid if best practice guidelines for treatment are followed. The BPT for fragility hip fracture is made up of a base tariff and a conditional payment, payable if a number of characteristics are achieved (e.g. time to surgery within 36 hours from arrival in an emergency department, or time of diagnosis of an admitted patient, fracture prevention assessments (falls and bone health, etc.); two Abbreviated Mental Tests (AMT) performed; and all the scores recorded in the National Hip Fracture Database (NHFD) with the first test carried out prior to surgery and the second after the stay (Van de Voorde et al., 2013). The Audit Commission's analysis for hip fracture shows that over time the base (non-BPT) tariff for hip fracture has decreased (and so has become punitive, in order to incentivise BPT uptake), whilst the BPT component price has grown. There were differences in the uptake of BPTs, which may be attributable to the different payment structure for each BPT (Gershlick, 2016a).

Figure 3.3. Pricing best practice tariffs, England (United Kingdom)

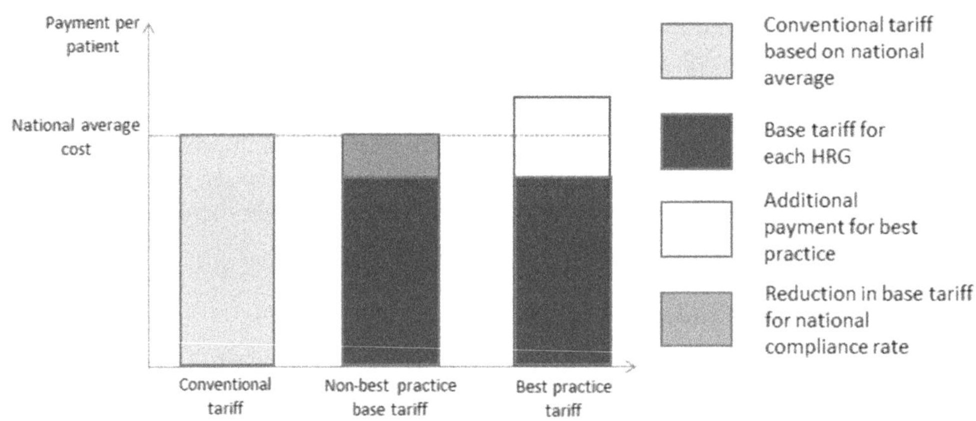

Source: Department of Health (2010).

In Sweden, the bundled payment for spine surgery includes a payment from intervention up to two years follow-up. It includes a warranty payment that pays upfront for potential complications and follow-up care (Bergauser Pont, 2014). Historical costs were used to inform price setting of the bundled payment rate. The tariff was comprised of several payments with up to 10% of the reimbursement being related to how functional the patient was one year after the surgery.

In the Netherlands, the bundled payment (which did not include a performance component) for diabetic patients defines a single annual payment per patient for all standard diabetic care. In 2010, the rates charged under the bundled payment contracts varied widely, from EUR 258 to EUR 474 per patient per year (Struijs et al., 2010). In 2011, fees started to converge, from EUR 381 to EUR 459 (Struijs et al., 2012a). The price differences were explained in part by actual differences in the care provided.

Outcomes gaining importance

Sweden's five-year pilot for hip and knee replacement incorporates health outcomes as part of the bundled payment. For spine surgery, the reform replaces the existing payment of global budget and DRG with a bundled payment where 10% of the payment is related to patient's functionality post-surgery. This is an innovative approach because a patient reported outcome measure is used to assess the extent to which the surgery succeeded in reducing back pain. The seven other conditions that are currently under development intend to use outcome measures in the payment. Sweden's well-developed quality registers are drawn on to inform how payments will be updated to better reflect value.

The initiatives in Sweden are closely related to the work conducted by the International Consortium for Health Outcomes Measurement (ICHOM) which was recently established as a non-profit organisation. Patients and physicians are involved in identifying outcomes which could lead themselves to robust measurement and comparisons (referred to as Standardised Sets of Outcomes). The Standard Sets of Outcomes can be used for different purposes in health systems: engaging with patients and discuss treatment options, systematically measuring outcomes; and using outcome information to purchase on value. Sets of Outcomes have been defined for twelve conditions including coronary artery disease, and low back pain. Components of the outcomes can include acute complications, patient-reported outcomes, disease reoccurrence in the case of back pain. By 2017, ICHOM aims to have published 50 Standard Sets covering more than 50% of the global disease burden (ICHOM, 2015).

The increased focus on outcomes in a number of bundled payment initiatives is not only related to tariff setting. It is still necessary to monitor outcomes when payments are bundled to ensure that providers do not cut corners. Early bundled payment contracts for diabetes care in the Netherlands contained only limited provisions for justifying the content and quality of care to health insurance companies but these provisions became increasingly important in newer contracts. Contracts now specify the obligations of the care group to provide the insurer with performance indicators for both processes (for example, the percentage of patients who had foot examinations in the previous twelve months) and outcomes (for example, the percentage of patients whose blood sugar levels are under control) (de Bakker et al., 2012).

In this respect, knowledge on the ways to best monitor quality is also evolving. A recent suggestion for diabetes care in the Netherlands recommends that indicators could better account for process along with outcomes to monitor quality (Struijs et al., 2012a). One approach would be to combine the information on process and outcome indicators into "linked indicators" where for example the percentage of patients having HbA1c levels above a certain threshold (outcome variable) and having undergone fewer than four standard diabetic check-ups in the past 12 months (process variable) could shed light on specific aspects of the quality of care (Voorham et al., 2008; Sidorenkov et al., 2011; Struijs et al., 2012a).

For Parkinson's disease in the Netherlands, a quality measuring effort preceded the payment reform (Figure 3.4). An agreed list of indicators applicable to care provided in outpatient hospital clinics was implemented in the neurology department of a select number of Dutch hospitals in 2014. In 2015, reporting on this indicator set became mandatory in all hospitals in the Netherlands.

Figure 3.4. Pilot for quality measurement for Parkinson's disease, the Netherlands

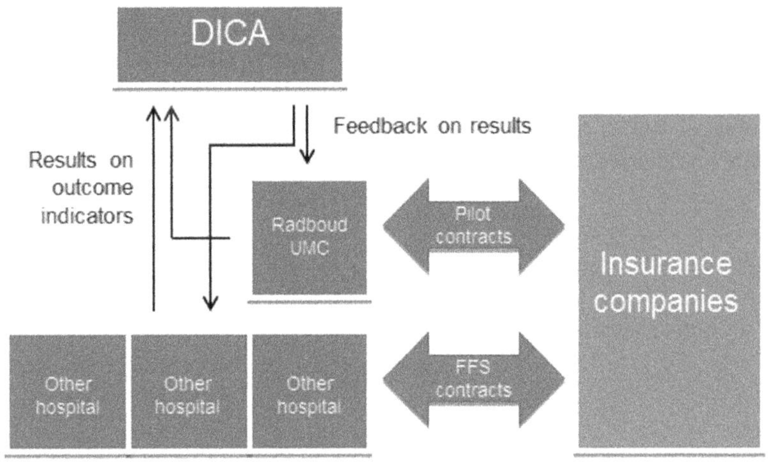

Source: Vlaanderen et al. (2016).

3.7. Building blocks for designing bundled payment

The case studies presented in this chapter reflect different approaches to bundled payment, in particular i) including pre or post-operative activities into care episodes; ii) incorporating quality elements into tariffs or reflecting costs of evidence-based care; and iii) defining single tariffs for chronic conditions. Each approach comes with specific challenges. Additionally, the limited evidence so far does not allow for a final verdict whether innovative bundled payments will drive up health system performance. Nevertheless, as set out below, there are some key lessons to draw from the country examples on the design and implementation of a bundled payment model. Policy attention should focus on conditions for implementation: the basket of services, setting tariffs, quality, stakeholder involvement, IT systems, and accountability.

Basket of services

The decision to include or exclude activities in bundled tariffs needs to be based on clear, transparent criteria. This also applies to the selection of the patient population the bundled payment should be applied for and whether high-risk patients are included. Episode-based bundled payments have clearer end points which may make monitoring easier. For chronic conditions, multiple bundle payments for patients with co-morbidities will have implications for how to handle their interaction. As the number of bundled payments increase for patients with multiple co-morbidities, alternative payment models may need to be considered.

Tariffs

Setting tariffs require historical data but it is important to be mindful of the bundled tariff level compared to previous levels. Where clear clinical guidelines exist, they can inform tariff setting as well as contribute to standardising protocols and mitigate payer concerns regarding transparency of a bundled payment approach.

Quality

Collecting data on quality should be built into the payment design – even if quality measures are not directly related to tariffs, they are still valuable for reporting purposes. Knowledge on ways to monitor quality is evolving – including data on outcomes. Data collection not only lays the foundation for monitoring, evaluation, and feedback but also brings about wider health systems changes for delivery with a more patient-centered approach.

Stakeholders

Irrespective of whether the move towards bundled payment is provider, purchaser or policy led, it is necessary for there to be shared joint aims and motivation among key stakeholders to achieve buy-in, particularly for mitigating diverging financial interests.

IT systems

IT system capability and adaptability to record bundled payment information is necessary. Ideally, making use of existing data and reporting requirements as much as possible is a good starting point to minimise administrative burden. It is necessary to mitigate administrative burden with data entry including the need for additional resources if a new system is implemented for staff training, and IT system compatibility with the bundled payment model, particularly for billing purposes.

Accountability

Monitoring, evaluation and feedback loops for reporting should be encouraged. Assessment of the impact of bundles payment should be embedded into the process with independent evaluation carried out on a systematic basis.

3.8. Conclusion

Bundled payments for acute care episodes that go beyond DRG, and for chronic conditions, are increasingly popular in a number of OECD countries. Initially including additional pre- or post-operative activities but limited to the inpatient sector, more sophisticated recent innovations foresee bundled payments that follow the patient across settings. Starting with bypass surgery in the early 1990s, the scope of inpatient care episodes for which bundled payment is applied has widened to include now a number of different clinical areas, in particular cardiac or orthopaedic procedures such as knee and hip replacement or spine surgery. Another recent trend is to set the tariffs of the bundled payment on the basis of best practice along an evidence-based pathway which increases transparency instead of simply reflecting the average costs of care provision. For chronic conditions, a small number of countries have started to implement bundled payments for either high prevalence conditions such as diabetes or low prevalence but high cost conditions such as HIV and Parkinson's disease.

Bundled payments based on best practice or adjusted according to quality indicators show some promise to achieve quality gains as illustrated in the country examples both for episodes-of-care and chronic conditions. The (limited) evidence presented in this chapter suggests that bundled payment appears to work better for improving quality in some areas than in others. For acute conditions, a number of initiatives have seen reductions in readmission rates, complications and improved mortality figures for hip and knee replacement and bypass surgery. For other procedures, such as stroke, experimentations have not shown any quality improvements. In the case of chronic conditions, better performance and higher patient satisfaction have been detected in the Netherlands for diabetes and Parkinson's disease and better adherence to medication and treatment protocol were associated with the bundled payments for HIV.

With regards to costs, a number of bundled payment initiatives have generated savings for payers. In the United States for example, Medicare as well as private sector innovations were able to reduce costs for bypass surgeries and hip and knee replacements, mainly achieved by reductions in average length of stay and reduced number of readmissions. For bundled payments for chronic conditions, average treatment costs for HIV were reduced in Portugal through better adherence to treatment plans but costs increased in the case of diabetes patients after the introduction bundled payments in the Netherlands which may be partly be driven by delaying required specialist care – not included in the bundled tariffs.

Whether the bundled payment will generate savings or even work also depends on local market conditions. It may work in places where providers have options to choose who they work with, or where it is mandatory, or where they are provider led or policy led. For example, differences in the participation of payers and providers have not been a deterrent in countries such as Portugal, England and the Netherlands. In Portugal and the Netherlands, provider participation was voluntary but mandatory in England. Payer participation was mandatory in England and Portugal but voluntary for insurers in the Netherlands. Payment reform was part of broader reforms in England and Portugal but this was not the case in the Netherlands, where changing the delivery of care was led by health professionals. More generally, this is a lesson for care networks and on how to operate in addition to policy considerations for bundled payment reform.

Bundled payments shift some of the financial risk of service delivery onto providers. This needs to be taken into account when identifying the clinical areas where bundled payments should be implemented, the services that should be covered by the bundled payment, the price of the tariffs and whether high-risk patients should be excluded from this payment scheme. The greater exposure to financial risk for providers is also a reason that negotiations about bundled payments between payers and providers can be challenging.

On the other hand, payers have concerns around transparency of payments when services are bundled. At any rate, very clear guidance is needed on defining bundles and for the services to be covered by bundled pricing arrangements. This seems to be less problematic for episodes-of-care which have clearer start and end points than for chronic conditions.

Evidence-based approaches can help support the development of services part of a bundle that draw on clinical guidelines to develop standardised sets of care and increase transparency, particularly when efforts focus on stakeholder engagement throughout implementation. In the initiatives analysed, providers mainly accepted and supported the introduction of bundled payments. Patients supported the eventual accompanying changes in the care delivery process but may not necessarily have been aware of the change in the mode of payment.

As is the case for other payment reforms, the introduction of bundled payments may present a trade-off between decisions based on clinical guidance and the provider's financial incentives if the bundled payments tariffs translate into reduced provider income as compared to the payment under the previous regime. Financial incentives for the more expensive hip replacement procedure led to greater uptake in England than in Scotland where financial incentives were not in place (Papanicolas and McGuire, 2015). Appropriateness criteria could also help guide bundle definitions to better support clinical decisions (Weeks et al., 2013).

There are further practical issues with bundled payments that need consideration. Bundled payments require sophisticated IT systems that can identify all services that are included in the bundled tariff. If claims data are not able to clearly identify services part of the bundle, this payment mechanism has its drawbacks. This was the motivation behind the CMS in the United States recently changing the rules of bundled payment to remove payment for post-operative visits from surgical packages. This was in part because the number of visits seemed to fall short of what was recommended. The removal from the package will allow for better monitoring of post-operative activity but it is unclear how surgeons will respond (e.g. more surgeries or see patients more often after surgery) (Mulcahy et al., 2015).

The CMS demonstrations of bundled payment models (part of the wider health reforms in the United States) are currently underway and so evaluations are not yet available. In the most comprehensive bundled payment model, there are important considerations related to volume and treatment. One study suggests that there are differences in spending growth for certain episodes suggesting that individual updates to payment rates for each episode may be appropriate but as the number of episodes expands, though, more systematic approaches to updating payment rates will likely be required (Rosen et al., 2013).

Policy makers should consider support tools needed to implement new payment methods alongside existing IT systems including software compatibility but also for staff so they are appropriately prepared and trained. They should also consider better systems for monitoring of payments.

In a number of countries, increased administrative burden related to bundled payments were reported. Some of the increased burden was related to collecting quality-related information as part of the introduction of bundled payments. Particularly in the case of bundled payments for chronic conditions, additional administrative problems can arise for patients with co-morbidities. For these patients health providers may have to manage the billing of services according to more than one pricing system. Clear standards for record keeping and reporting would help mitigate some of the issues raised in the country examples. That said, for the treatment of multi-morbid patients, bundled payments geared towards only chronic condition may be of limited success and alternative more comprehensive payment models may be more effective such as population-based payments (see Chapter 4).

Bundled payments can profit from the increased popularity of patient outcome measurement in a number of countries. These measures show potential to better inform and incentivise payments in some areas of health care delivery. Wider system effects may better align health policy priorities with payment policies in the long run towards more patient-centered care with greater emphasis on evidence-based guidelines and using outcomes to inform price setting and payment.

Note

1. Medicare Part A covers mainly inpatient hospital stays and limited rehabilitative care whereas Part B covers physician and nursing care, hospital outpatient services and other services such as diagnostics and laboratory tests.

References

Beersen, N. et al. (2011), "Onderzoek naar de meerwaarde van ParkinsonNet".

Berghauser Pont, L. (2014), "A Case-based Study on Value Based Reimbursement for Spine Surgery and Potential Implementation in the Netherlands. Learning from the Swedish Health Care Innovations in Value Based Reimbursement for Spine Surgery", Master's Thesis.

Berry, S.A. et al. (2009), "ProvenCare: Quality Improvement Model for Designing Highly Reliable Care in Cardiac Surgery", *Quality and Safety in Health Care*, Vol. 8, No. 5, pp. 360-368, http://dx.doi.org/10.1136/qshc.2007.025056.

Bloem, B.R. and M. Munneke (2014), "Revolutionising Management of Chronic Disease: The ParkinsonNet Approach", British Medical Journal, Vol. 348.

Calsyn, M., J.D. Ezekiel and J. Emanuel (2014), "Controlling Costs by Expanding the Medicare Acute Care Episode Demonstration", *JAMA Internal Medicine*, Vol. 174, No. 9, pp. 1438-1439.

Casale, A.S. et al. (2007), "ProvenCareSM: A Provider-driven Pay-for-performance Program for Acute Episodic Cardiac Surgical Care", *Annals of Surgery*, Vol. 246, No. 4, pp. 613-621.

Darzi, A. (2008), "High Quality Care For All – NHS Next Stage Review", Department of Health, London, https://www.gov.uk/government/uploads/system/uploads/attachment_data/file/228836/7432.pdf.

de Bakker, D.H. et al. (2012), Early Results from Adoption of Bundled Payment for Diabetes Care in the Netherlands Show Improvement in Care Coordination", *Health Affairs*, Vol. 31, No. 2, pp. 426-433, http://dx.doi.org/10.1377/hlthaff.2011.0912.

de Bruin, S.R. et al. (2013), "Quality of Diabetes Care in Dutch Care Groups: No Differences Between Diabetes Patients With and Without Co-morbidity", *International Journal of Integrated Care*, Vol. 13, pp. 1-12.

de Lau, L.M. and M.M. Breteler (2006), "Epidemiology of Parkinson's Disease", *The Lancet Neurology*, Vol. 5, No. 6, pp. 525-535, http://dx.doi.org/10.1016/S1474-4422(06)70471-9.

Delbanco, S. (2014), "The Payment Reform Landscape: Bundled Payment", *Health Affairs*, Blog 2 July 2014, http://healthaffairs.org/blog/2014/07/02/the-payment-reform-landscape-bundled-payment/.

Department of Health (2016), "England Case Example – Maternity Pathway", unpublished, submitted for the OECD Project on Payment Systems.

Department of Health (2010), "NHS Payment by Results – Guidance for 2010-11", London.

Dutch Healthcare Authority (2014), "Market Scan and Policy Letter Healthcare Insurance Market", Dutch Healtcare Authority, Utrecht.

Gershlick, B. (2016a), "England Case Example – Best Practice Tariffs", submitted for the OECD Project on Payment Systems, http://www.oecd.org/health/paying-providers.htm.

Gershlick, B. (2016b), "England Case Example – NHS Long Term Care 'Year of Care' funding model", unpublished, submitted for the OECD Project on Payment.

Hasaart, F. (2011), "Incentives in the Diagnosis Treatment Combination Payment System for Specialist Medical Care. A study about behavioural responses of medical specialists and hospitals in the Netherlands", University of Maastricht.

Hussey, P.S., M.S. Ridgely and M.B. Rosenthal (2011), "The PROMETHEUS Bundled Payment Experiment: Slow Start Shows Problems In Implementing New Payment Models", *Health Affairs*, Vol. 30, No. 11, pp. 2116-2124.

ICHOM (2015), "Standard Sets", http://www.ichom.org/medical-conditions, accessed 1 June 2015.

IMPAQ International (2013), "Evaluation of the Medicare Acute Care Episode (ACE) Demonstration: Final Evaluation Report", IMPAQ International, Colombia, United States, http://downloads.cms.gov/files/cmmi/ACE-EvaluationReport-Final-5-2-14.pdf, accessed 2 June 2015.

Ivbar Institute (2015), "Swedish National Development of Value-based Models", http://www.ivbar.com, accessed 19 June 2015.

Lee, T.H., A. Bothe and G.D. Steele (2012), "How Geisinger Structures its Physicians' Compensation to Support Improvements in Quality, Efficiency and Volume", *Health Affairs*, Vol. 31, No. 9, pp. 2068-2073.

Lourenço, A. (2016), "Portugal Case Example – Bundled Payment Per Patient Treated", submitted for the OECD Project on Payment Systems: http://www.oecd.org/health/paying-providers.htm.

Marshal, L., A. Charlesworth and J. Hurst (2014), "The NHS Payment System: Evolving Policy and Emerging Evidence", Research Report, Nuffield Trust, London.

McDonald, R. et al. (2012), "A Qualitative and Quantitative Evaluation of the Introduction of Best Practice Tariffs", Evaluation Report commissioned by the Department of Health, University of Nottingham.

Mechanic, R. (2011), "Opportunities and Challenges for Episode-Based Payment", *New England Journal of Medicine*, Vol. 365, pp. 777-779.

Mulcahy, A.W. et al. (2015), "Medicare's Step Back from Global Payments – Unbundling Postoperative Care", *New England Journal of Medicine*, Vol. 372, No. 15, pp. 1385-1387.

Munneke, M. et al. (2010), "Efficacy of Community-based Physiotherapy Networks for Patients with Parkinson's Disease: A Cluster-randomised Trial", *The Lancet Neurology*, Vol. 9, No. 1, pp. 46-54.

Nelson, L. (2012), "Lessons from Medicare's Demonstration Projects on Value-Based Payment", *CBO Working Paper 2012-02*, https://www.cbo.gov/sites/default/files/WP2012-02_Nelson_Medicare_VBP_Demonstrations.pdf.

Nijkrake, M.J. et al. (2010), "The ParkinsonNet Concept: Development, Implementation and Initial Experience", *Movement Disorders*, Vol. 25, No. 7, pp. 823-829.

Nolte, E. and C. Knai (2014), "Approaches to Chronic Disease Management in Europe", in E. Nolte, C. Knai and R.B. Saltman (eds.), *Assessing Chronic Disease Management in European Health Systems – Concepts and Approaches*, European Observatory Study Series No. 37, World Health Organization.

Papanicolas, I. and A.J. McGuire (2015), "Do Financial Incentives Trump Clinical Guidance? Hip Replacement in England and Scotland", Seminar Office of Health Economics, London, https://www.ohe.org/events/do-financial-incentives-trump-clinical-guidance-hip-replacement-england-and-scotland#sthash.seRQM98C.dpuf.

Patel, K. et al. (2015), "Transforming Oncology Care: Payment and Delivery Reform for Person-Centered Care", *American Journal of Managed Care*, May, http://www.ajmc.com/journals/issue/2015/2015-vol21-n5/Transforming-Oncology-Care-Payment-and-Delivery-Reform-for-Person-Centered-Care.

Paulus, R.A., K. Davis and G.D. Steele (2008), "Continuous Innovation in Health Care: Implications of the Geisinger Experience", *Health Affairs (Millwood)*, Vol. 27, No. 5, pp. 1235-1245.

Porter, M., C.M. Marks and Z.C. Landman (2014a), "OrthoChoice: Bundled Payments in the County ofStockholm (A)", Harvard Business School Case.

Porter, M., C.M. Marks and Z.C. Landman (2014b), "OrthoChoice: Bundled Payments in the County of Stockholm (B)", Harvard Business School Case.

Raaijmakers, L.G. et al. (2013), "Perceived Facilitators and Barriers in Diabetes Care: A Qualitative Study Among Health Care Professionals in the Netherlands", *BMC Family Practice*, Vol. 14:114, http://www.biomedcentral.com/1471-2296/14/114.

Ridgely, M.S. et al. (2014), "Bundled Payment Fails to Gain a Foothold in California: The Experience of the IHA Bundled Payment Demonstration", *Health Affairs*, Vol. 33, No. 8, pp. 1345-1352.

Rosen, A.B. et al. (2013), "Policy Makers Will Need a Way to Update Bundled Payments that Reflects Highly Skewed Spending Growth of Various Care Episodes", *Health Affairs*, Vol. 32, No. 5, pp. 944-951.

Rudkjøbing, A. et al. (2015), "Evaluation of a Policy to Strengthen Case Management and Quality of Diabetes Care in General Practice in Denmark", *Health Policy*, Vol. 119, No. 8, pp. 1023-1030.

Sidorenkov, G. et al. (2011), "Review: Relation between Quality-of-care Indicators for Diabetes and Patient Outcomes: A Systematic Literature Review", *Medical Care Research and* Review, Vol. 68, No. 3, pp. 263-289.

Struijs, J.N. and C.A. Baan (2011), "Integrating Care through Bundled Payments – Lessons from the Netherlands", *New England Journal of Medicine*, Vol. 364, No. 11, pp. 990-991.

Struijs, J.N., J.T. van Til and C.A. Baan (2010), "Experimenting with a Bundled Payment System for Diabetes Care in the Netherlands: The First Tangible Effects", National Institute for Public Health and the Environment, Bilthoven, http://www.rivm.nl/bibliotheek/rapporten/260224002.pdf.

Struijs, J.N. et al. (2012a), "Three Years of Bundled Payment for Diabetes Care in the Netherlands: Impact on Health Care Delivery Process and the Quality of Care", National Institute for Public Health and the Environment, Bilthoven, http://www.rivm.nl/bibliotheek/rapporten/260013002.pdf.

Struijs, J.N. et al. (2012b), "Effects of Bundled Payment on Curative Health Care Costs in the Netherlands: An Analysis of Diabetes Care and Vascular Risk Management Based on Nationwide Claim Data", National Institute for Public Health and the Environment, Bilthoven, http://www.rivm.nl/dsresource?objectid=rivmp:188652&type=org&disposition=inline&ns_nc=1.

Thorsen, T. (2008), "General Practice Reception of the Coordination Fee for Diabetes Patients – A Qualitative Evaluation After the First Year [Almenpraksis' modtagelse af forløbsydelsen for diabetespatienter – Enkvalitativ evaluering efter det første år], Synthese onbehalf of Fagligt Udvalg og Dansk Almenmedicinsk Kvalitetsenhed(DAK-E), Copenhagen.

Thorsen, T. (2007), "Forløbsydelsen – et feasibility study med særligt fokuspå praksis med mange sårbare patienter" [Fee for diabetes patients – A feasibility study with a focus on practices with many vulnera-ble patients], *Forskningsenheden for Almen Praksis* [Section ofGeneral Practice]. University of Copenhagen.

Tsai, T.C. et al. (2015), "Medicare's Bundled Payment Initiative: Most Hospitals Are Focused on a Few High-Volume Conditions", *Health Affairs*, Vol. 34, No. 3, pp. 371-380.

Van de Voorde, C. et al. (2013), "A Comparative Analysis of Hospital Payments in 5 Countries", Health Services Research (HSR), Belgian Health Care Knowledge Centre (KCE), KCE Reports 207. D/2013/10.273/61, Brussels.

van der Marck, M.A. et al. (2013), "Integrated Multidisciplinary Care in Parkinson's Disease: A Non-randomised, Controlled Trial (IMPACT)", *The Lancet Neurology*, Vol. 12, No. 10, pp. 947-956.

Vlaanderen, F.P. et al. (2016), "Netherlands Case Example: The Dutch Outcome-based Payment Model of ParkinsonNet: A Case Study", submitted for the OECD Project on Payment Systems, http://www.oecd.org/health/paying-providers.htm.

Voorham, J. et al. (2008), "Cross-sectional Versus Sequential Quality Indicators of Risk Factor Management in Patients with Type 2 Diabetes", *Medical Care*, Vol. 46, pp. 133-141.

Weeks, W.B. et al. (2013), "The Unintended Consequences of Bundled Payments", *Annals of Internal Medicine*, Vol. 158, No. 1, pp. 62-64.

Welikala, J. (2014), "Bedford Refuses to Sign Circle MSK Contract", *Health Service Journal*, 7 November.

Wensing, M. et al. (2011), "Connectedness of Healthcare Professionals Involved in the Treatment of Patients with Parkinson's Disease: A Social Networks Study", *Implementation Science*, Vol. 6:67.

Wohlin, J. et al. (2016), "Effects of Introducing Bundled Payment and Patients' Choice of Provider for Elective Hip and Knee Replacements in Stockholm County", Medical Management Centre Karolinska Institute, Stockhom.

Chapter 4

Population-based health care provider payments

This chapter discusses population-based payment to pay groups of health providers – referred to as Accountable Care Organisations (ACOs) in the United States and elsewhere. ACOs are financially accountable for the provision of all or the vast majority of health care services to a defined population. They are permitted to keep part of the savings they generate provided they meet specific quality criteria.

A number of initiatives have been carried out in recent years. The assessment reveals positive outcomes in a number of cases. Care strategies depend on the provider composition and the characteristics of the population they are financially accountable for. The ability to generate savings depends on the extent provider groups are able to identify and effectively manage high-cost and at-risk patients. However, caution must be exercised in generalising preliminary results because of the large differences in the technical design of ACOs as they operate in different environments.

4.1. Overview

Payments that cover all – or the vast majority of – health care services for a defined group of the population takes the concept of bundled payment a step further. Unlike the innovations described in Chapter 3, population-based payments are not limited to specific care episodes or chronic conditions. This *population-wide approach* is rooted in the conviction that bundled payments for *selected* chronic conditions may not sufficiently address care issues around multi-morbid patients, and in particular the elderly. Population-based payments are made to groups of health providers such as independent primary care physicians, specialists, practice networks, hospitals or nursing homes as well as management companies, which might be partially owned by health providers. The main motivation behind this form of payment is the apparent failure of traditional payment systems to overcome fragmentation of care. Siloed payments tied to care delivery by separate providers are seen as detrimental to effective integration of care. Population-based payments aim to enable care integration by readjusting the principal objectives of paying for health care: instead of paying *providers,* money follows the *patients* across providers; and instead of paying for treatment of episodes of one *disease*, a more holistic view of the *well-being* of the population is taken.

The innovative aspect of population-based bundled payment generally lies in the prospect for providers to share some of the savings that they are able to generate for the payers in case they can reduce treatment costs while meeting pre-defined quality requirements. In practical terms, this means that population-based payments define a prospective budget for a population and providers are financially rewarded if they can keep total costs below the benchmark value. The financial arrangements can also foresee that provider groups bear the risk of financial losses when total costs exceed this value. In most cases however, the actual payment for individual services continues to be done via traditional payment mechanisms such as FFS, but the benchmark budgets act as an incentive to keep costs down.

In a number of countries, capitation payments are no new phenomenon: managed care initiatives have been tried before to shift financial risk onto providers. In the United States, in the 1980s and 1990s these set out capitated contracts to a network of providers to manage a defined population. In the United Kingdom, in the 1990s, GP fundholding contracts which included specific hospital care; drugs; staffing in the practice; and community services had similar characteristics. Although managed care contracts in the United States have helped to bring costs down in the early stages this was soon followed by the "managed care backlash". Providers were unhappy with the lower prices they initially agreed on with Managed Care Organisations and were able to negotiate more favourable terms as provider markets consolidated (Frakt and Mayes, 2012). Patients complained about required pre-authorisation and other restrictions that many of their Managed Care plans entailed which in some cases led to denial of care (Frakt and Mayes, 2012; Barnes et al., 2014). A major difference between capitation under Managed Care contracts and the new population-based payments is that the former did not bear any incentive to improve or just ensure a minimum level of health care quality. The innovative developments presented in this chapter frequently include provisions to make sure that quality targets are met. Thus, they initiate a shift away from exclusively paying for *volume* to reward *quality improvements* and *efficiency gains*.

These payment reforms can be considered as one pillar towards a more effective integration of care activities. The implementation of population-based payments, the definition of the population, the services provided by the groups of health providers and their strategy to reduce costs while improving quality differs between health systems and needs to be analysed within the country context. This chapter first presents a number of examples of recently-implemented population-based payment schemes. Then, it compares their impact on quality and costs, as well as the conditions for their implementation, before analysing some important technical aspects in more detail. Finally, some key challenges associated with these innovations are discussed.

4.2. Population-based payment innovations are currently implemented in a variety of countries

Population-based payment is closely related to the emergence of so-called Accountable Care Organisations (ACO) in the United States and elsewhere. ACOs are groups of health care providers that are collectively accountable for the organisation of health care and its quality and also take the financial responsibility of care provision. In some countries, population-based payment contracts can also be signed with non-health care providers such as management companies and other private contractors. ACOs *do not* act as health insurers – the ACOs themselves do not sell any health plans to the population. They rather contract health insurers (or other payers) and guarantee the provision of health care for their insured population for a predefined budget. ACOs are responsible for the delivery of all – or the vast majority of – health care services for a defined group of the population. The largest experiments currently happen in the United States where around 400 ACOs are contracted by Medicare. Another 200 ACOs have negotiated population-based payment contracts with private insurers. In total, ACOs in the United States provide care for about 20 million patients (Shortell et al., 2014a). Smaller initiatives exist in Germany, for example in a rural area in South-Western Germany with a physician-led ACO and in the Spanish region of Valencia where a private contractor is accountable for primary and secondary care in several health areas.[1] In Hungary, a population-based payment model existed between 1998 and 2008 but its implementation was deprioritised and the model finally discontinued in the wake of discussions around the privatisation of parts of the SHI system (Gaál et al., 2011). Similar concepts are currently piloted or discussed in a number of additional countries including Singapore, New Zealand, the Netherlands and Portugal.

Strong political commitment for Medicare ACOs in the United States

In the United States, Accountable Care Organisations (ACOs) are part of broader reforms of the Affordable Care Act (ACA) of 2010. One aim of this reform is to change payment under Medicare to move away from a strict FFS scheme paying health providers for increasing activity towards a payment system rewarding quality and efficiency. There is strong political commitment to tie at least 30% of Medicare payment to quality or value through alternative payment models by 2016 and 50% by 2018 (Burwell, 2015). One of the alternative payment models are population-based payments to ACOs. The ACA mandated CMS to contract ACOs for the care of a defined population of Medicare patients.

Medicare ACOs require a minimum population of 5 000 patients. Providers forming an ACO typically include primary care providers and hospitals but can also extend to specialists, long-term care facilities, and home care. ACOs must commit to participate in the Medicare programme for at least three years, develop a formal structure that allows the organisation to receive and distribute payments for shared savings, include a sufficient number of primary care providers, establish a leadership and management structure that includes clinical and administrative systems, define processes that promote evidence-based medicine and patient engagement, report on quality, cost measures and care co-ordination mechanisms and demonstrate that the ACO is patient-centered (Shortell et al., 2014a).

First implemented in 2012, three types of Medicare ACO programmes are currently operating (CMS, 2015a):

- Medicare Shared Savings Programme (MSSP) ACO,
- Advanced Payment ACO, and
- Pioneer ACO.

The programmes designed by CMS differ in the extent to which savings are shared between ACOs and Medicare and the financial risk assumed by the ACOs. For all models, savings can only be earned when quality targets are met. The largest programme is the Medicare Shared Savings Programme where the vast majority of ACOs have shared-saving-only contracts. In the Advance Payment initiative, Medicare makes upfront payment to rural ACOs with less access to capital. The upfront payments are consolidated with later savings. The Pioneer ACO model is the most integrated and demanding one. CMS only contracted organisations to this arrangement which had previously proven to be able to effectively manage health care across providers. In the first two years of contract, Pioneer ACOs share gains and losses with Medicare but with a higher level of reward and risk than ACOs under the MSSP. In the third year, Pioneer ACOs that have realised savings in the previous two years can move towards a prospective monthly capitation payment. Thus, they assume a higher financial risk but have bigger flexibility in spending. The Pioneer ACOs are also encouraged to start negotiating value-based models of health care delivery with other payers outside Medicare, such as Medicaid and private insurers.

The alternative quality contract for the private sector in Massachusetts

The Commercial Health Insurer Blue Cross Blue Shields in Massachusetts (BCBSMA) proposed a change in payment for groups of providers as part of their Alternative Quality Contract (AQC) from 2009 onwards. BCBSMA has roughly 2.8 million policy holders. Groups of providers eligible to sign the AQC must include primary physicians and they must collectively care for at least 5 000 people enrolled in BSBSMA Health Maintenance Organisation (HMO) and Point-of-Service (POS) plans. In 2009, eight provider groups signed the AQC with BCBSMA. The eight provider groups encompassed around one fourth of all primary care physicians in the BCBSH HMO and POS network and one third of all patients in these networks. The AQC contract length was five years (Chernew et al., 2011).

The AQC foresaw a virtual global budget with shared savings and losses for the provider groups. In 2009 and 2010 the AQC also included additional payments for quality improvements. As of 2011, AQC made shared savings dependent on quality performance.

Total virtual budgets and annual increases are negotiated between BCBSMA and provider groups individually, taking past spending for patients as a starting point. The budget is risk-adjusted annually to take account of changes in patient's health status. The virtual budgets cover all health care services – with the exception of mental health and substance abuse treatment – delivered to patients, irrespective whether the services were provided by a member of the provider group or not. Provider groups are required to have re-insurance for exceptional expensive patients. The actual services throughout the year are billed on a FFS basis but are reconciled at the end of the year with the virtual budget. From 2011 on, increases of the virtual budget were linked to a regional spending benchmark.

Establishment of a private ACO in Northern California to compete for patients

In Northern California the commercial insurer Blue Shields of California, the independent practice association Hill Physicians and the hospital system Dignity Health collaborated in an ACO to compete for clients with the integrated care system Kaiser Permanente. In 2010, the three parties concluded an ACO contract for 41 000 insurees belonging to the California Public Employees' Retirement System (CalPERS) in Sacramento. The four main goals of the ACO were to:

- Keep CalPERS as a client for Blue Shields (and hence for the providers) by guaranteeing zero cost and premium growth in the first year;
- Attract new public agencies to contract with CalPERS (and hence with the ACO);
- Maintain or improve quality of care; and
- Create a sustainable business model for extension to other regions.

The partners agreed on a number of strategies and initiatives to keep costs down and improve quality such as better exchanges of patient medical information, co-ordinated clinical processes and comprehensive home-based medical care for high-risk patients and the elderly.

Blue Shields and providers agreed on a virtual global budget with upside and downside risk-sharing savings and losses. Seven cost categories were defined, and costs per month per member were stipulated and, for each cost category, the risk for over – and under-spending were allocated between the parties (Markovic 2012).

After a predominantly successful implementation of the ACO model in Sacramento generating significant savings and some quality improvements, each of the parties concluded additional ACO contracts either with the same or other partners in other regions. The IPA Hill Physicians, for example, is currently engaged in four commercial ACO contracts covering 72 000 out of their 300 000 patients (The Commonwealth Fund, 2014).

Physician-led joint venture in South-Western Germany contracted by two health insurance funds

In 2006, two statutory health insurance funds – AOK Baden-Württemberg and LKK Baden-Württemberg – contracted a private joint venture "Gesundes Kinzigtal GmbH" (GK) to run a population-based integrated care model with a virtual budget and one-sided risk sharing in a rural area in South-Western Germany (Milstein and Blankart, 2016).

A network of doctors owns two-thirds of GK and a health management company (Optimedis AG) owns the remaining part. In 2012, GK had contracts with 86 providers including: GPs, outpatient specialist, hospitals nursing homes, physiotherapists, pharmacies (Hildebrandt et al., 2012). Providers contracted by GK are paid by health insurers in the traditional way (e.g. FFS) while there are separate payments from GK for services outside the benefit package (e.g. maintaining and update electronic health record) and to set up an IT infrastructure. Those doctors that are co-owners of GK (via their share in the doctor's network) participate additionally in any financial success of GK. These additional payments amount to 10-15% of provider income (Llano, 2013). Duration of the contract is ten years.

Currently, about one third of 31 000 eligible patients participate voluntarily in this model. They can end their participation on a quarterly basis. There are only very small financial incentives for participants such as vouchers for gyms or co-payment reductions, but enrollees benefit from tailored prevention and sports programmes (Milstein and Blankart, 2016).

A virtual budget is based on the existing risk-adjusted capitation amount the two health insurers receive from the Central Health Fund as part of the risk-structure compensation scheme. Potential savings are calculated as the difference between the virtual budget and the actual cost of the whole population insured with the two health insurers in the region. The virtual budget refers to the entire insured population and not only the participating patients to prevent any kind of risk selection by GK. Earned savings for GK are not related to explicit quality targets but as the model is based on voluntary participation of patients, the provision of low quality health care can indirectly affect the potential to earn savings if patients decided to end their participation in the model.

After showing some success in reducing spending growth and improving quality the model is now being replicated in other parts of the country. A critical mass of patients appears to be crucial to effectively manage care in a region but given the nearly 118 statutory health insurers in Germany, such a concentration is rare and seems to be essential for the success of the model in the German context.

A public-private partnership as a starting point for accountable care in Spain

Legal changes allowed for the establishments of public private partnerships (PPP) in the health sector in the late 1990s in Spain. The first PPP was implemented in the region of Valencia. There, the regional Health Ministry established a PPP for ten years with a private contractor (Ribera Salud Group) which required the contractor to construct a hospital and manage hospital care in one health area in Valencia (Alzira) covering 245 000 patients that are automatically enrolled. In return, the contractor received annually adjusted capitation payments. The contract was changed in 2003 to cover primary and secondary care services and its duration extended to 15 years. Health care is organised around one hospital, two outpatient clinics and 30 health centres (Acerete et al., 2011).

Under the current contract, the annual capitation payment is adjusted in line with the regional health budget. The contract stipulates that possible profits of the private contractor are to be shared between contractor and local government; contractors can keep profits up to 7.5% of turnover but must return any additional profit in excess of it. The fixed capitation payment also covers investment costs for medical and non-medical equipment which is under the responsibility of the contractor. However, after expiration of the contract, the equipment becomes property of the regional administration. People in the health area are automatically assigned to the contractor without enrollment, but if they choose health care outside the health catchment area then Ribera Salud has to assume 100% of the costs incurred. To assure high-quality treatment, health providers of Ribera Salud have to meet a series of targets covering a wide range of quality and safety objectives including process indicators, clinical outcomes and patient experience.

The model has meanwhile spread to other health areas of Valencia. In 2011, around 20% of the population of Valencia was covered under similar contracts (NHS European Office, 2011).

Moving towards population-based payments in additional countries

Similar population-based care integration models are currently implemented or piloted in a number of other countries.

In ***Singapore***, several programmes were launched in recent years especially targeted at the elderly and frail population (McClellan et al., 2014). The Singapore Programme for Integrated Care for the Elderly (SPICE) is a community-based initiative using local care centres and home care to enable elderly patients to be cared for in the community rather than in hospitals. The Holistic Care for Medically Advanced Patients (HOME) targets palliative care for patients with end-stage heart, lung, liver and renal failure. These care models are partially funded by capitated monthly payments to health providers enabling them to pool these funds. Aged Care Transition teams facilitate the patient's transition to the optimal care setting facilitating the delivery of co-ordinated care after hospital discharge. First evaluations of outcomes are positive. The SPICE programme has reduced the number of emergency department visits by 50% and the HOME programme has helped increase the number of patients who choose palliative care in their homes instead of hospitals after struggling with fatal diseases. Aged Care Transition teams have prevented 17 000 hospital days per year, saving USD 11 million annually (McClellan et al., 2014).

In ***New Zealand***, 20 county district health boards are responsible for financing and provision of health and disability services for the population within their district. One of these district boards is Counties Manukau Health (CMH) near the city of Auckland caring for more than 500 000 people (Alderwick et al., 2015). With funding allocated by the government, CMH has to purchase most primary care services and provide hospital-based and specialist services. Primary care is predominantly provided by Primary Health Organisations (PHO); they are networks of self-employed GPs, nurses and other health professionals. PHOs receive an adjusted capitation payment from the district health boards for every enrolled patient. CMH has alliance agreements with the five PHO partners operating in its district stipulating shared system-wide responsibility and integration across community and hospital care providers. Since 2013, the district alliance agreement between CMH and the five PHO includes some financial risk and gain sharing (NZ Doctor, 2013). The agreement stipulates that savings generated from reduced costs in emergency departments in one of the hospitals of CMH will be redistributed to the PHOs. On the other hand, PHOs will be penalised if a patient visit to an emergency department could have been served in a PHO.

The Netherlands has piloted efforts to move in the direction of population-based payments. In 2013, nine care groups[2] were piloting different initiatives in population health management ranging from better co-operation between primary care and secondary care to projects fostering more cost-effective prescribing and improved care for mental health. A number of projects were also geared towards the elderly population with an enhanced discharge management after hospitalisation, screening for dementia, loneliness and polypharmacy and proactive engagement of geriatric nurses to identify particularly vulnerable patients (RIVM, 2014). Patient involvement in the development of these population management initiatives is high. They are represented via patient advocacy groups in eight of the nine pioneer sites. So far, the pilot projects have been funded by different payers such as health insurers or via research grants from public organisations. There are plans to implement the population health management initiatives in purchaser-provider contracts with shared savings similar to the type of Alternative Quality Contract (AQC) as seen in the private sector in the United States. However, there are ongoing discussions to what extent the Dutch health system is flexible enough to incorporate this new payment approach or whether there are some legal or regulatory obstacles impeding this development.

In ***Portugal***, the creation of Local Health Units in 1999 (ULS – *Unidade Local de Saúde*), a group of NHS providers, was a move towards vertical integration between primary care and hospital services within the same geographical area. ULS have centralised management and have co-ordinated services between both hospitals services and primary health centres. This model of care intends to improve multi-disciplinary co-operation between different levels of care to achieve efficiency gain and provide more patient-centered care. Since 2010, ULS are predominantly financed through risk-adjusted capitation adjusted to reflect population characteristics which gives the ULS greater financial and operational freedom to experiment with innovative care delivery models. In 2014, there were eight USL in Portugal (OECD, 2015a). Recent evaluations show cost savings in maternity care and primary care diagnostics and some evidence of lower volume of hospital activity. The ULS model has not reached maturity yet as it has scope to further improve co-ordination of care in more areas of service delivery and to further innovate (OECD, 2015b).

Besides the new payment models targeted at ACOs presented in this chapter, there exist a number of fully integrated health systems, such as Kaiser Permanente that also share some similarities with ACOs. The main difference between these integrated systems and an ACO is that the former frequently combine the function of insurance and health provision. Moreover, policy holders with Kaiser Permanente health care coverage typically have to stay within their network of providers for treatment. Payments to or within these integrated systems is outside the scope of this chapter.

Framework to compare the impact of payment reform and conditions for implementation

Table 4.1 gives an overview of early assessments of the impact of reforms that promote population-based payments in the United States, Germany and Spain and describes the conditions for their implementation in more detail. The United States have a huge variety of ACO models – three types of Medicare ACO models and various ACO models from the private sector. Findings for the United States draw from the evaluation of the Medicare models, the AQC model rolled out by a private insurer in Massachusetts and a Sacramento ACO contracted by one private insurer. For Germany, results are drawn from one ACO (the joint venture GK), the findings from Spain are based on several ACOs in the same region which are operated by the same management company (Ribera Salud), frequently referred to as the Alzira model.

Table 4.1. Assessment and implementation conditions for population-based payment in three countries

	United States	United States	United States	Germany	Spain
Type and name of payment reform	Medicare ACO	AQC Massachusetts	ACO Sacramento	Population-based bundling (GK)	Population-based bundling (Alzira)
Assessment of policy impact					
Achievement in terms of policy objective :					
Quality	+/-	+	+/-	+	+
Savings	+/-	+/-	+	+	+
Other					
Unintended consequences	Best performing ACO can lose revenues		Increase in emergency department visits		Contract renegotiation
Conditions for implementation					
Payment reform embedded in larger policy reform	+			+	+
Stakeholder participation in policy development (e.g. actively consulted in establishment of law/scheme)					
Payer participation	Mandatory for Medicare	Voluntary	Voluntary	Voluntary for SHI funds	Mandatory for public payer in some regions
Provider participation	Voluntary	Voluntary	Voluntary	Voluntary	Voluntary
Administrative Burden	+				+
Data collection and use	New and existing data			New and existing data	
How are tariffs set?	FFS embedded in benchmark based on past spending and adjusted annually for total Medicare spending trend	FFS embedded in negotiated benchmark	FFS embedded in negotiated benchmark	FFS embedded in benchmark based on SHI funds reimbursement from risk-structure equalisation	Negotatied capitated amount, adjusted annually with total regional health budget increase
Independent evaluation of reform	+	+	+	+	-

Source: Authors' compilation.

4.3. Assessment of payment reforms

In many cases in the United States as well as for GK in Germany, the introduction of population-based payment to ACOs was pursuing the *Triple Aim* (Berwick et al., 2008) of:

- improving population health,
- improving health care quality and patient experience, and
- reducing health care costs.

To achieve these aims, ACOs have to rethink and redesign the pathway of care delivery focussing on patient needs and improve co-operation between providers. They need to identify areas where savings can be generated, for example, by reducing double examinations and by providing care more efficiently in a less costly setting. Quality and outcomes can be enhanced if care pathways are streamlined and follow best practice or evidence-based guidelines and if variation in practice can be reduced.

The implementation of population-based payment is relatively recent. Evaluations of possible improvement in health outcome, quality of care and reductions in spending draw on data available over a few years at best and need to be considered preliminary at this stage. Moreover, any effect of the introduction of population-based payments typically cannot be isolated as it closely connected to a change in the organisation of care and the process of care delivery that accompanies the establishment of an ACO. Restructuring care processes across providers takes time to bear fruit. Thus, a more robust assessment of the potential success of this payment innovation will require a longer time horizon.

Many ACO achieve quality improvements with regards to process, only few for outcome

There are some indications that quality of care is increasing when provided by ACOs in the United States. Within the Medicare programme, all 32 Pioneer ACO could successfully report the required 33 quality measures in their first year and overall these ACOs were reporting a higher level of performance than for benchmark Medicare beneficiaries for 15 available clinical indicators. Around three-quarters of them reported lower readmission rates when compared to the Medicare beneficiaries' benchmark. In their second year, the Pioneer ACOs were able to improve their performance in 28 of the 33 quality measures, for example for controlling high blood pressure, screening for future fall risk and screening for tobacco use and cessation. The greatest improvements could be observed for the at-risk population which suggests that Pioneer ACOs are making some progress in co-ordinating care for patients with chronic conditions (Kocot et al., 2014). Similar results are found for the much larger MSSP ACO programme within Medicare. An evaluation showed that patient experience was positive and care co-ordination for patients with chronic conditions for patients in the MSSP ACO programme had improved (McWilliams et al., 2014). Patients could access doctors more quickly, had better access to visit notes, and were better informed by their primary care physician about specialty care.

More time-robust findings exist for some longer-standing private ACOs. Over four years, improvements in quality were faster for those patients enrolled in ACOs contracted by BCBS for the AQC in Massachusetts than for a control group. This refers to a better performance in process measures for ambulatory care in the area of chronic disease management, adult preventive care and paediatric care as well as to intermediate outcome measures, such as blood pressure control (Song et al., 2014). For the private ACO in Sacramento, hospital readmissions within 30 days decreased by 15% in the first year (Markovich 2012). Over the same period though, emergency department utilisation increased.

Although no quality targets are set as part of the ACO contract in Germany, evaluations found reduced mortality rates for those persons participating in the ACO model, higher two-year survival rates for chronic heart disease patients, while a programme for the elderly showed improvement in nutrition behaviour but no improvement in physical activity and no changes in health-related quality of life. Patients treated by participating physicians had lower hospitalisation rates, and were more likely to be prescribed medicines according to evidence-based guidelines. Patients and providers appear to be satisfied with the programme (Hildebrandt et al., 2012; Mnich et al., 2013; Busse and Stahl, 2014).

Internal evaluations of the hospitals attached to Ribera Salud in the Spanish region of Valencia showed significantly better results compared to other hospitals in the same region. Waiting times for emergency visits and external consultations are half that of the regional average. Readmission rates and average length of stay are also substantially below average rates in the region. Patient satisfaction for patients treated by ACO-affiliated hospitals is very high and significantly above satisfaction rates in other hospitals (NHS European Office, 2011). But there are also reports about skimping of care for patients with chronic conditions such as HIV (Acerete et al., 2011).

ACOs contributed to slowing spending growth on an aggregate level but not all ACOs at the individual level reduced spending

On an aggregate level, ACOs in the United States have slowed Medicare health spending growth in recent years. But not all ACOs were able to generate savings, and among those that did, not all realised the minimum savings required to be eligible to keep part of the savings (CMS, 2013; CMS, 2014). Concerning the Pioneer ACOs, Medicare could generate net savings in both evaluated performance years. Spending growth per beneficiary assigned to Pioneer ACOs was below spending growth of similar Medicare beneficiaries in both years: 0.3% vs. 0.8% in 2012 and 1.4% vs. 1.85% in 2013. But in both years, less than half of participating ACOs generated enough savings to share the gains with Medicare (12 out of 32 in 2012, and 11 out of 23 in 2013). Some ACOs had to share "losses" with Medicare and for the rest of the Pioneer ACOs, actual costs were not significantly different from benchmark figures. As a result of the difficulties encountered in effectively managing financial risk, nine Pioneer ACOs dropped out of the programme after the first year. Results from the much larger MSSP ACO model showed that more than 50% of all ACOs reduced health spending growth in the first year (118 out of 220), but only a quarter (52) were entitled to keep and distribute part of the savings to their members. In total, they were allowed to keep USD 315 million in 2012. For Medicare, the total net savings from MSSP ACOs amounted to USD 383 million. Payment innovations within the Medicare system – including population-based payments to ACOs – have been identified as a contributing factor to the recent slowdown in US health spending growth rates (White House, 2014).

Evaluations from private sector ACOs contracted by the AQC model of BCBS in Massachusetts covering a longer time period show that saving on claims compared to the control groups were realised in each of the four years. However, BCBS did not generate savings in the first three years as the savings on claims were below the top-up payments (e.g. shared savings, quality bonuses, infrastructural support) integrated in the model. Net savings for the payer could only be recorded in the fourth year and are due to reduced prices and reduced utilisation on outpatient care, imaging and tests (Song et al., 2014). The private ACO in Sacramento was able to reduce cost in its first year against projected spending based on past trends but also in absolute terms compared to the previous year. Spending went down by 1.6% while spending in the control group increased by 9.9%. Over two years, the annual spending growth rate per member in the ACO was around 3% which was significantly below the spending growth that the insurer (Blue Shields of California) experienced elsewhere in the state. Thus, one of the main aims of the Sacramento ACO – the slowdown of insurance premium increase for the California Public Employees' Retirement System (CalPERS), a major client of insurer and the provider groups – was achieved. Over three years, the accumulated savings in insurance premium payment by CalPERS beneficiaries stood at USD 59 million or USD 480 per member per year (Markovich, 2012; The Commonwealth Fund, 2014).

In 2012, the German GK had a virtual budget of EUR 68.6 million with the health insurer AOK and realised savings of around EUR 4.6 million which meant that actual costs were 6.6% below the benchmark budget (Gesundes Kinzigtal, 2014). On a per capita basis, AOK received EUR 141 more from the Central Health Fund than it actually spent for the patients in the region. Comparing billing data of GPs participating in the ACO model with those that do not, it was found that cost increase per patient was significantly lower for participating GPs (+7%) than for non-participating GPs (+19%) over the period 2006 to 2010 (Hildebrandt et al., 2012).

In Spain, internal evaluations of Ribera Salud publish very large savings for the ACO in the health area of Alzira, with costs 25% lower than the average cost per inhabitant in Valencia (EUR 607 vs. EUR 825 in 2010) but no external validation are available to confirm these figures (NHS European Office 2011). However, the success story of this ACO model is questioned in other reports which claim that savings are overestimated as the capitated payment received by the Ribera Salud excludes a number of cost items included in the regional benchmark figure (Acerete et al., 2011).

A number of unintended consequences observed for some ACOs

In a number of instances, the establishment of ACOs around population-based payments brought about some unintended consequences. In Spain, the first population-based contract in the Valencia region signed in 1999 which only related to secondary care was financially not viable for the contractor Ribera Salud. It was modified in 2003 by the regional ministry to include primary care resulting in an increase in the capitation rate. This contractual change was interpreted by some as a bail-out by the regional government for an unsustainable business model (Acerete et al., 2011). Renegotiating contracts is not an uncommon issue with public-private partnerships and public payers are often in a delicate position to give in to demands to private contractors if they do not want to compromise the provision of vital public services. There are also reports about staff dissatisfaction with working conditions in hospitals managed by Ribera Salud in Spain which may be due to reduced wages and deteriorating working conditions and skimping of care for some groups of chronic patients (Acerete et al., 2011).

In the context of the Medicare ACOs, Toussaint et al. (2013) report that even well-performing ACOs can be confronted with reduced total revenues despite gaining savings from Medicare. The best performing Pioneer ACO in the first year (Bellin ThedaCare Health Partners ACO serving an area in Wisconsin) recorded a reduction in total revenues in their first year. This was due to the fact that only 18% of their patients were covered under the ACO Medicare payment model with the remaining 82% being covered under traditional FFS schemes from private insurers and Medicaid. However, the improved care processes they implemented as part of the ACO Model also benefitted patients covered under other schemes whose payment contracts did not foresee a possibility to earn savings. Consequently, an avoided hospital admission for a traditional FFS patient translated into less revenue for the ACO. Hence, Medicare encourages Pioneer ACOs to implement additional shared savings contracts with other payers to counterbalance any possible revenue reduction. There are also some unintended consequences with regards to quality: the Sacramento ACO was successful in reducing hospital admissions and readmission in their first year but at the expense of increased use of emergency departments.

4.4. Conditions for implementing payment reform

Population-based payment innovation part of wider policy reform and piloted before larger roll-out

Implementation of population-based payments has gained traction in all countries because the payment reform was frequently part of a wider health policy reform. In the United States, the creation of Medicare ACOs was included in the ACA of 2010. ACOs are considered as one important tool to move away from a strict FFS scheme towards a payment system that rewards quality and value for Medicare beneficiaries. Other alternative modes of value-based payments – such as bundled payments or pay-for-value programmes for hospitals and physicians are also tested.

In Germany, the establishment of the joint venture GK as an ACO and its payment via a shared-savings contract was an example of an "Integrated Care Contract". Integrated care contracts between individual insurers and individual providers were made legally possible in the early 2000s. They permit selective contracting between individual health insurance funds and individual or groups of providers promoting care integration across health sectors. Modes of payment and models of care can be negotiated between the contracting parties (Milstein and Blankart, 2016). In Spain, the implementation of the ACO model followed a change in national law to allow for a PPP in the health sector in the late 1990s.

Roll out of the new model of payment and care provision started gradually in the United States. The different types of Medicare ACOs were phased in slowly in 2012 starting initially with a low number of ACOs. But many of their features were already tested before in earlier programmes such as the Physician Group Practice Demonstrations (PGP). The PGP was a Medicare programme carried out between 2005 and 2010 for ten practice groups bringing together 5 000 physicians providing care for 220 000 Medicare beneficiaries. The positive experiences of this programme facilitated the implementation of Medicare ACO concept. For Germany, the GK can be considered as a pilot and the management company co-owning GK is currently planning to establish similar arrangements in other regions. The Alzira Model in Spain has meanwhile been scaled up and by 2011 the Ribera Salud Group had implemented six population-based contracts in different areas of the region of Valencia.

The history of the private sector ACOs in the United States was sometimes less driven by a broader policy change. The Sacramento ACO was created by an insurer (Blue Shields of California), an independent practice association (Hill Physicians) and a hospital system (Dignity Health) in Northern California for predominantly economic reasons, as a tool to keep costs down in a competitive environment. The three parties agreed to collaborate in an ACO out of concerns of Blue Shields of California that one of their biggest clients – the California Public Employees' Retirement System (CalPERS) might switch their health coverage to Kaiser Permanente. As Kaiser Permanente is a fully integrated health system, this move would also have affected Hill Physicians and Dignity Health because these providers would have no longer been able to serve patients with a Kaiser Permanente health plan.

Voluntary participation for provider and patients in ACO can encourage take-up

In all countries, participation in the new payment model is voluntary for providers. In the United States, different health providers can freely decide to form an ACO and apply to Medicare for inclusion in the ACO programme. In the private sector, providers need to agree with commercial insurers on ACO contracts. In the German example, the contract is negotiated between insurers and a joint venture comprised of health providers and a management company. In Spain, contract negotiations take place between private contractors and regional health ministries. For payers, engagement in these types of payment models is also voluntary with the exception of the United States where Medicare is mandated to offer several legally defined payment models to ACOs but they select the participating ACOs. Patients have some choice as well. Medicare patients can choose freely among doctors that accept Medicare payments. However, patients themselves do not decide whether they participate in the ACO or not. They are "assigned" to an ACO by Medicare if their doctor participates. Same can be true for private sector ACOs in the United States. Within the German ACO framework, patients have to be actively registered but they can end their participation at any time. In Spain, patients are automatically assigned to a primary health centre run by the ACO but they are free to choose specialist care in hospitals not managed by Ribera Salud.

Investments in IT infrastructure vital for ACO

The existence of a sophisticated IT infrastructure seems to be a crucial factor in the eventual success of an ACO. In particular, bringing health care costs down requires good case management and the stratification of patients to identify those who benefit most from early interventions. The extent to which IT is used in the management of an ACO will depend on several factors, most importantly the level of service integration. Analysing a variety of examples, McClellan et al. (2013) find that the most successful arrangements use integrated IT systems that allow real-time monitoring of metrics. This requires inter-operational IT systems with universal patient records being accessible by various providers collaborating in an ACO. These IT systems can also include decision support mechanisms and direct interaction within the clinical work flow. They appear to be particularly effective when connected to registries and public reporting systems. On a less advanced level, electronic management of appointment and referrals may help reduce waiting times and improve case management. IT support is also required for the collection and submission of data to calculate quality indicators which are required in different ACO programmes in the United States as well as in Spain. Finally, stratification of patients to identify those who benefit most from early interventions also requires constant monitoring of a number of patient-specific parameters at a central level. In the case of the Spain, the ACOs are the frontrunners in the use of IT: the hospitals associated with Ribera Salud in Valencia were reported to be the first public hospitals with a fully integrated electronic medical history system including medical notes, test results and imaging (NHS European Office, 2011).

But setting up the appropriate IT infrastructure is expensive. This is why in some cases either the payer (Medicare in the case of the advanced ACO model) or the ACO itself (e.g. the German GK) supports participating health providers financially with the acquisition and installation of the required IT infrastructure.

Considerable administrative burden for some ACOs

The management of shared savings contracts can come with considerable administrative burden for participating providers. This can be due to contract managing, the measurement and reporting of cost and quality indicators which are drawn from existing or new data or intensified case management. The level of administrative burden ultimately depends on the environment an ACO operates in and the care strategy adopted by an ACO. These issues seem to be most pronounced in the United States. ACOs or the participating providers are frequently engaged in more than one risk-sharing contract. ACOs that are contracted by Medicare in the Pioneer ACO programme are actually encouraged to engage in similar contracts with other payers such as Medicaid or private insurers. The independent practice association Hill Physicians – which is one contracting party in the Sacramento ACO – is currently involved in three additional ACOs. For each payer, important elements of the ACO contracts can differ, be it the risk-sharing models, the minimum saving requirements, the benchmarking budget or the quality indicators which make contracting management a complex endeavour. Addicott and Shortell (2014) report that one health provider network engaged in four different ACO arrangements was required to report on 219 different performance measures. Consequently, the need for different payers to agree on a common set of quality of cost measures has been identified as one of the key issues to dominate the discussion on the future of ACOs in the United States (Shortell et al., 2015). In Spain, the establishment of a public private partnership contract in the health sector and its eventual re-negotiation appears to have been a rather complex endeavour. But unlike in the United States, the ACOs in Spain are only contracted by a single payer. In addition to the administrative burden imposed by contracting payers, the internal management of the ACO may also entail some administrative activities, such as facilitating the communication between all participating providers.

Past spending important element in defining benchmark values

Providers continue to be paid for the provision of services in the traditional way in all population-based payment models, which is mainly FFS in the case of US Medicare ACO programme and private ACOs as well as in Germany. The Spanish contractors receive capitation payments to provide primary and secondary care. Whether providers can get any additional financial reward generally depends on their ability to keep the costs below a benchmark budget. There is some variety in the way these benchmarks are set in the different models and a number of important technical features need to be considered when defining these benchmarks.

Total health costs of the ACO are mapped against these target values to determine whether the ACO has generated savings or losses. In the Medicare model and in Germany, these values are based on administrative data and rules with no additional negotiations. For Medicare ACOs, the benchmark values are calculated individually based on the weighted average expenditure per ACO beneficiary over the past three years, adjusted for beneficiary characteristics. It is inflated with annual average Medicare cost growth rate for future years. In Germany, the benchmark is defined annually by the Central Health Fund via the Risk-Structure-Compensation mechanism[3] automatically. The benchmark for GK corresponds to the amount of money the two contracted health insurers receive from the Central Health Fund.

Moving to the private sector in the United States, the benchmark values as well as their annual increases for ACOs with AQC from BCBSMA were the result of individual negotiations. The starting point was typically historic spending levels as the intention was to control future cost increases rather than reduce the initial budgets of ACOs. Consequently, provider groups with higher initial spending were granted lower annual increases than ACOs with lower costs. As of 2011, annual spending increases were tied to regional spending benchmarks (Song et al., 2014). In the Sacramento ACO, benchmark values and annual changes were agreed upon by all contracting parties with the overall aim to keep Blue Shields premiums for CalPERS policy holders low. In Spain, the first capitation fees (including only hospital care) were negotiated between Ribera Salud and the regional ministry of health. Initially, annual increases were linked to the consumer price index. After reshaping the model which resulted in higher negotiated capitation (including also primary care), the annual growth was tied to the yearly increase in the regional health budget.

Population-based payments initiatives are frequently accompanied by independent evaluation

An independent evaluation of the impact of reforms in payment mechanisms or service delivery is generally considered conducive to the overall acceptance by providers and patients. Moreover, it should provide policy makers with unbiased information on the success of a reform. The Medicare ACO programmes are regularly evaluated by independent researchers and results publically available. An independent consultant also analysed the early impact of the Sacramento ACO. In Germany, evaluations are co-ordinated by an institute attached to the medical department of a university. In Spain, however, the impact of the ACO model on costs and quality of care has not been evaluated by an independent authority.

4.5. Population-based payment and ACO models differ in important technical aspects

After summarising the general impact of population-based payment on the quality and costs of care and some issues around their implementation, a more technical discussion related to the composition of ACOs and the financial arrangements is useful to better understand how they work in practice. Table 4.2 displays the most important contractual features of the five population-based payment models and ACO types analysed in this chapter.

Table 4.2. Technical characteristics of some population-based payments to ACOs

	ACO examples				
	United States			Germany	Spain
ACO criteria	Medicare*	AQC*	Sacramento	GK	Alzira
Population size	>5 000	>5 000	41 000	9 400	245 000
Lead provider	Main types: hospital-lead, physician-led, joint hospital-physicians	Main types: hospital-lead, physician-led, joint hospital-physicians	Joint hospital group and independent practice association	Network of primary care physicians, outpatient specialists and management company	Hospital (managed by private contractor)
Payment	Most: FFS with benchmark budget; few Pioneer ACO: capitation	Most: FFS with benchmark budget	FFS with benchmark budget	FFS with benchmark budget	Capitation with benchmark budget
Contract type	Shared savings and risk, some only shared saving	Shared saving and risk (between 50-100%)	Shared saving and risk	Shared saving	Shared saving and risk
Contract duration	3 years	5 years	Not specified	10 years	15 years
Setting of benchmark	Based on past ACO spending, adjusted annually for total Medicare spending trend	Negotiated individually, taking into account each ACOs baseline spending	Negotiated global budget based on per member-per month allowable costs across seven cost categories	Virtual budget: defined by SHI risk-structure equalisation scheme	Capitation: initial negotiation, adjusted annually with budget increases
Assignment of population	Retrospectively	Prospectively	Prospectively	Not relevant	Prospectively
Financial accountability	All Medicare Part A and B spend for assigned population	All health care for HMO and POS patients with some exceptions	Total health care costs	All SHI cost for population living in the area	Total spending of regional MoH with some exceptions
Risk contract	Shared savings beyond threshold; higher rate of saving if two-sided contract	Unpublished	Different risk sharing profiles for hospital group, practice group and insurer for different cost categories	Unpublished; roughly 50-50 between payer and ACO for every EUR	Savings beyond 7.5% back to MoH
Incorporation of quality	Shared savings can only be gained if quality requirements are met; earned savings function of performance	In 2010 and 2011: additional payments based on quality indicators; since 2012 shared savings only if quality requirements are met	No explicit quality requirements, but quality monitored by contracting parties	No explicit quality requirements, but quality monitored by contracting parties, and incorporated through competition with standard care	Quality indicators must be met as part of contract

* The ACOs Medicare and AQC are programmes open to different individual ACO models which differ in some of their characteristics.

Population size and provider composition differ between and within countries

The size of the population that is prospectively or retrospectively assigned to an ACO varies widely between countries reflecting differences in multi-payer and single-payer health systems as well as the size of the pool of providers involved and differences in care organisation and delivery process. In the United States, the population size of ACOs generally ranges between 5 000 and 50 000. In Spain, 245 000 inhabitants of the health area Alzira are automatically assigned to the ACO. It is not clear whether there is an optimal population size of an ACO to be successful, but it needs to be high enough for the care organisation to pool patient risk. In the context of the Medicare programme, analysing early results of the MSSP ACO after the first year showed that small, predominantly physician-led ACOs with fewer than 8 000 patients generated savings for Medicare which may indicate that smaller ACOs can implement changes in the delivery of care more quickly (McClellan et al., 2015). In case important investments in new care delivery methods are made, bigger populations may be required to create economies of scale. Analysing the whole landscape of ACOs in the United States, Shortell et al. (2015) conclude that a minimum size of 25 000 to 50 000 enrollees would be needed to refinance needed investments.

There is also some variety with regards to the composition of providers organised within an ACO. The provider composition of an ACO will strongly influence the care strategy the ACO will implement to reduce spending and improve care quality. In Germany, the ACO is composed of a network of primary care physicians and outpatient specialists, and a management company. Other providers such as in secondary care are part of a wider network and have contractual agreements with GK. In Spain, Ribera Salud organises its ACO model around a hospital in the Alzira area. In the United States, a great variety exists, both in the public and private sector. Analysing a first survey of existing ACOs around eight key characteristics including size, scope of health services provided, and degree of integration, Shortell et al. (2014b) clustered ACOs into three categories:

- Large systems with a high degree of integration delivering a wide range of services frequently including one or more post-acute facilities,
- Smaller physician-led practices, which are centered around primary care, delivering a much narrower range of services,
- Medium-sized, joint hospital-physician and coalition-led groups that offer a moderately broad scope of services with some involvement of post-acute facilities.

ACOs prefer shared saving with some risk sharing embedded in traditional payment system

One aim of population-based payment is to incentivise groups of providers to reduce total growth of health care costs. In practice, this is done by defining a benchmark value as a target budget incorporating total health care costs – or the cost for the vast majority of health services – for the defined population assigned to the ACO. In case patient costs remain below this benchmark value, the ACO and payer share the savings. In some models, ACOs have to reimburse part of their payment to the payer in case the costs are above the benchmark. The actual mode of payment frequently remains FFS and total costs will be compared and reconciled with the target budget at the end of the year. Thus, financial risk of care provision is partially shifted from payers to providers in these payment models. In general, three main contract types can be distinguished:

- Shared savings contract (one-sided risk contract) embedded in FFS payment regime,
- Shared saving and risk contracts (two-sided risk contract) embedded in FFS payment regime,
- Capitation payment (with full risk or risk-sharing contract).

The majority of the Medicare MSSP ACOs and the German GK have one-sided risk contracts protecting them from possible negative financial consequences if they overspend. However, the management of the German GK is financed exclusively out of savings, so the profitability of the model is vital. Only few Medicare MSSP ACOs but all Pioneer ACO have two-sided risk contracts. This is also true for the AQC contracts of Massachusetts and the Sacramento ACO in the private sector. In Spain, Ribera Salud receives a capitation payment but it needs to share any savings if profits exceed 7.5% of turnover. For Medicare, moving from paying individual providers by FFS to monthly capitation for the ACOs is also a strategic aim for the most advanced Pioneer ACOs.

The shared savings and risk contracts usually have duration of multiple years which give all contracting parties some planning security. Developing innovative care strategies and re-shaping patient management and care pathways to bring costs down might also take some years to bear fruit. In some instances, ACO have important up-front investment for IT infrastructure or equipment to support innovative care models. In these cases, allowing

ACOs to recuperate their investment by accumulating gained savings over a longer time period appears to be necessary. Within the Medicare programme, ACOs commit for three years. The Alzira contract in Spain has the longest duration with 15 years as the private contractor was required to finance the construction of a hospital which is the lead provider of this ACO model.

ACOs are accountable for different populations and different services

The monetary benchmark value for ACOs with shared savings contracts is defined by the *size of the population* and the *range of health services* they are accountable for. With regards to the *population*, their financial responsibility in most cases corresponds to the population assigned to the ACO. For Medicare, the population is assigned *retrospectively* depending on whether a Medicare patient received the vast part of their primary care services from a provider working within an ACO in that year. In the private sector in the United States, patients are assigned *prospectively* based on their insurance policy. This means that ACOs know in advance the population they are financially responsible for. The same is true in Spain where Ribera Salud receives capitation payments for the automatically assigned population. The situation is different in Germany. There, GK is not only financially accountable for the population that is actively enrolled in the ACO model but the *entire* population of the two contracted insurers in the region. Currently, only around one third of them are enrolled.

The different ACO models also vary in the *range of health care services* they are financially responsible for. In the Medicare model, the benchmarks reflect Medicare Part A and B health care costs, which essentially reflect inpatient hospital care, some skilled nursing care, hospice and home health services as well as outpatient care and doctor's services. In private ACOs, financial responsibility typically reflects all costs for services they are contractually obliged to provide. In Massachusetts' AQC, costs for mental health and substance abuse treatment are outside the benchmark budget. In Spain, the capitation payment reflects costs for primary care and secondary care. The budget does not include costs for outpatient pharmacy, oxygen therapy, prosthetics and transport (Acerete et al., 2011). In Germany, the benchmark cost reflects nearly all services borne by the Statutory Health Insurance, including primary care, hospital care, post-acute care but also dental care and pharmaceuticals. Long-term care is not included. In some population-based payment models, adjustments are made in the calculation of total costs to exclude outlier costs for exceptionally expensive patients. In many cases, ACOs are financially accountable for a wider range of services than directly delivered by the provider group forming an ACO.

Hence, the benchmark budgets the ACOs are held accountable for are defined by the size and characteristics of the population and by a range of services which vary between the different ACO models. These factors will have an influence on provider group's strategies to reduce total spending growth.

Providers and payers both seek benefits from reduced spending growth

Population-based payment contracts between payers and ACOs are a tool used to control health spending growth by letting payers and provider groups share the savings generated by innovative care models. In some contracts, the contracting parties also share potential losses. Beyond these very broad characteristics, shared savings/loss contracts have to define a number of important details when implemented. Analysing the design and application of a sample of ACOs in the United States, Weissman et al. (2012) identify some basic properties with regards to measurement and distribution of savings to be included in a risk contract, mainly to limit the risk of payers. These are:

- Inclusion of a risk threshold or minimum savings rate,[4]
- Starting point of shared savings,[5]
- Distribution cap or maximum pay-out,
- Distribution of savings *between ACO and payer*,
- Distribution of savings *between individual providers* forming an ACO.

For Medicare patients, the savings contracts differ whether the ACO participates in a one-sided or two-sided risk contract (CMS, 2015b). In the one-sided model, ACOs are eligible to share savings up to 50% (depending on quality performance) above the minimum savings rate – set between 2% and 3.9% of the benchmark costs based on the size of the assigned population. Total savings are capped at 10% of the benchmark costs.

In the two-sided model Medicare model, ACOs are eligible to share savings up to 60% (depending on quality performance) above the minimum savings rate – set at 2% of the benchmark costs. Total savings are capped at 15% of the benchmark costs. Losses only have to be repaid when costs exceed the benchmark value by 2%. The share of losses ACO have to carry is calculated as 1 minus the shared savings rate but cannot exceeding 60%. Losses are capped at 5% of benchmark value in the first year, at 7.5% in the second year and 10% in the third year.

Less detailed information is available for other ACO contracts. For the private sector, Weissman et al. (2012) conclude that in those cases where shared savings contracts include risk thresholds, these lie between 2 to 5% of the benchmark value. Providers are typically allowed to keep between 20 to 80% of the savings. The contract for the ACO in Sacramento is more detailed. It stipulates different risk distributions for specific health care components between all contracting partners based on the extent to which insurer and providers can influence the costs (Table 4.3).

In Germany, savings are shared roughly 50/50 between GK and insurers without a minimum savings rate. In Spain, there exists a pay-out cap of 7.5%. All profits generated by Ribera Salud beyond this threshold have to be returned to the regional government.

Table 4.3. Allocation of risk for the three partners in the Sacramento ACO

	Share of risk if costs are above/below target value per cost category		
Cost category	Hospital group	Physician group	Insurer
Partner hospital	50%	25%	25%
Out-of-area non-partner hospital	25%	25%	50%
Other non-partner hospital	30%	30%	40%
Professional	30%	35%	35%
Mental health	0%	0%	100%
Pharmacy	33.3%	33.3%	33.3%
Ancillary	25%	25%	50%

Source: Adapted from Markovich (2012).

Little seems to be published on how the savings are distributed among providers forming an ACO. CMS does not stipulate how Medicare ACOs as legal entities have to distribute any savings among their members. Analysing some survey information on early

Medicare ACOs, Dupree et al. (2014) find there is variation between ACOs on how savings are distributed depending on the provider composition. In some cases, part of the gained savings will be retained at the ACO level to foster investment in infrastructure. When distributed to providers it seems that the biggest proportion will go to primary care physicians followed by specialists and other stakeholders. The distribution can also depend on performance and quality metrics. The distribution can also be decided on the basis of different costs categories, as is the case for the ACO in Sacramento (Table 4.2). In the German ACO model, around half of the net savings – after programme costs were retained by GK and used to finance further investments and the rest distributed among partners and the two owners of the joint venture (Die Zeit, 2015).

Quality a decisive factor in risk-sharing contract

Improving population health and quality of health care are two of the major goals of population-based payments. ACOs in the Medicare programme are required to meet a number of predefined quality standards to be eligible to share potential savings with CMS. Additionally, quality performance has an impact on the absolute amount of earned savings as it is included in the formula to calculate the shared savings ratio. In total, there are 33 quality measures which cover patient/care giver experience, care co-ordination/patient safety, preventive health and for some populations at risk such as for diabetes, hypertension, and ischaemic vascular disease, heart failure and coronary artery disease (see Table 4.4).

Whereas only the reporting of these indicators was sufficient to meet minimum quality requirements in the first year, the relative performance of an ACO with regards to these measures is taken into account from the second year on. For each indicator, a benchmark performance is calculated based on claims and quality data for FFS Medicare beneficiaries or Medicare Advantage plans. Points are awarded on a sliding scale. Minimum attainment level is set at 30% percentile of benchmark. The maximum score is awarded at the 90% percentile level (CMS, 2015c).

The AQC initiative in Massachusetts foresaw additional quality-related payments based on 64 indicators with half of them relating to care in hospitals and the other half to outpatient care in the first two years. The indicators were process measures, intermediary outcomes and patient experience and were combined in one metric with intermediary outcome measures having more weight. Quality incentive payments were outside the budget and providers could earn up to 10% of additional income. As of 2011, quality measurements are included in the shared savings contract with improved quality translating into a larger share of savings that can be retained by the ACOs.

Part of the ACO agreements in Spain is that hospitals meet a number of quality targets defined by the regional governments covering process indicators (e.g. waiting times), clinical outcomes (e.g. immunisation and morality rates) and patient experience (NHS European Office, 2011).

Table 4.4. Quality indicators used in the Medicare MSSP ACO programme

Domain	Measure	Description
Patient/Caregiver experience	ACO-1	Getting timely care, appointments and information
Patient/Caregiver experience	ACO-2	How well your doctors communicate
Patient/Caregiver experience	ACO-3	Patients' rating of doctor
Patient/Caregiver experience	ACO-4	Access to specialists
Patient/Caregiver experience	ACO-5	Health promotion and education
Patient/Caregiver experience	ACO-6	Shared decision making
Patient/Caregiver experience	ACO-7	Health status/Functional status
Care co-ordination/Patient safety	ACO-8	Risk standardised, all condition readmissions
Care co-ordination/Patient safety	ACO-9	Ambulatory sensitive conditions admissions: COPD or asthma in older adults
Care co-ordination/Patient safety	ACO-10	Ambulatory sensitive conditions admission: heart failure
Care co-ordination/Patient safety	ACO-11	Percent of PCPs who qualified for EHR incentive payment
Care co-ordination/Patient safety	ACO-12	Medication reconciliation
Care co-ordination/Patient safety	ACO-13	Falls: Screening for fall risk
Preventive health	ACO-14	Influenza immunisation
Preventive health	ACO-15	Pneumococcal vaccination
Preventive health	ACO-16	Adult weight screening and follow-up
Preventive health	ACO-17	Tobacco use assessment and cessation intervention
Preventive health	ACO-18	Depression screening
Preventive health	ACO-19	Colorectal cancer screening
Preventive health	ACO-20	Mammography screening
Preventive health	ACO-21	Proportion of adults who had blood pressure screened in past two years
At-risk population diabetes	Diabetes composite	ACO-22: Hemoglobin A1c Control (HbA1c) (<8%) ACO-23: Low density lipoprotein (LDL) (<100 mg/dL) ACO-24: Blood pressure (BP) < 140/90 ACO-25: Tobacco non use ACO-26: Aspirin use
At-risk population diabetes	ACO-27	Percent of beneficiaries with diabetes whose HbA1c in poor control (>9%)
At-risk population hypertension	ACO-28	Percent of beneficiaries with hypertension whose BP < 140/90
At-risk population ischemic vascular disease	ACO-29	Percent of beneficiaries with IVD with complete lipid profile and LDL control < 100mg/dl
At-risk population ischemic vascular disease	ACO-30	Percent of beneficiaries with IVD who use aspirin or other antithrombotic
At-risk population heart failure	ACO-31	Beta-blocker therapy for LVSD
At-risk population coronary artery disease	CAD composite ACO-32-33	ACO-32: Drug therapy for lowering LDL cholesterol ACO-33: ACE inhibitor or ARB therapy for patients with CAD and diabetes and/or LVSD

Source: Adapted from CMS (2015d).

Population-based payments incentivise ACOs to develop a wide range of strategies to keep health care costs down

In all countries, ACOs that succeeded in reducing costs while improving or maintaining quality of care developed a care strategy. This strategy heavily depends on the country-specific context, the composition of the providers forming an ACO as well as on the nature of the payer but also on the composition of the patients the ACOs are financially accountable for.

Most health care costs arise from the need of only few patients. Using data from the Medical Expenditure Panel Survey (MEPS) in the United States, Stanton and Rutherford (2005) estimate that 80% of the total health care costs stem from only 20% of the population and multi-morbid patients cost up to seven times as much as patients with a single chronic condition. For Medicare, the most expensive 10% of patients are responsible for 52% of total spending (De Nardi et al., 2015). The most promising strategy to generate savings for an ACO therefore lies in a stratification of patients and identifying patients at risk. For those, specific prevention programmes can be developed or case management intensified.

When developing its care strategy, the private sector ACO in Sacramento reviewed data of the 5 000 chronically ill patients that accounted for 75% of its costs. Based on this analysis it identified five key priorities: improving information exchange, the co-ordination of processes such as discharge planning, the elimination of unnecessary care, limiting variation of practice and reducing costs for pharmaceuticals (Markovich, 2012).

In successful ACOs, care models were rethought and pathways redesigned to make them more patient-centered with less fragmentation between the providers. Frequently, patients were included more in the decision process and empowered to play a more active role in the self-management of diseases. Case management of patients was strengthened and programmes to manage diseases adopted to reduce duplication of work and variation in treatment. Data exchange between providers improved with the establishment of electronic health records and tools enabling real-time data exchange.

Analysing a survey on the first wave of ACOs in the United States, Colla et al. (2014) found that over 50% of ACOs are physician-led with a further third being jointly led between physicians and hospitals. The survey also showed that physician-led ACOs are less likely to provide emergency, post-acute services and other services involving different providers as compared to ACOs under joint or other leadership. This could make it harder for physician-led ACOs to effectively manage the transition of patients between settings. On the other hand, physician-led ACOs are more likely to have comprehensive care management programmes in place and are more actively engaged in pre-visit planning, medication management and preventive care reminders (Colla et al., 2014; Shortell et al., 2015). In an analysis to assess to what extent surgeons are involved in the first wave of Medicare ACOs, Dupree et al. (2014) found that most ACOs focussed on improving care co-ordination for patients with chronic conditions and reducing hospitals readmission and emergency department visits. While ACOs which include hospitals tried to reduce hospital readmission to avoid financial penalties from Medicare, ACOs exclusively comprised of physicians focussed on reducing hospital admission and emergency department visits. Reducing unnecessary surgery does not appear to be a priority in the early years but could potentially be important in the future.

One example of how providers have actually reshaped care processes is that of the provider ThedaCare (Pioneer ACO) (McClelland et al., 2013). ThedaCare focussed on redesigning inpatient care. They set up interdisciplinary teams composed of nurses, physicians, care manager and pharmacists which meet with a patient right after admission. These teams create a uniquely tailored care plan with the nurse being responsible for monitoring progress and strict adherence to protocol. In addition, social workers meet with every patient to assess the need for home-based support. As a result, average length of stay has been cut by 17% and duplication of work reduced substantially. At the same time, patient satisfaction substantially increased.

Data for the private sector AQC model in Massachusetts show that savings in the outpatient sector were most significant (Song et al., 2014). Costs for procedures, imaging and test could be reduced and savings could be explained by a mix of lower prices and reduced utilisation. This could serve as an indication that ACOs contracted for the AQC model put their focus on the reduction of double examination and more targeted referrals.

The ACO in Sacramento developed a very clear strategy to achieve the substantial cost savings that they agreed upon already in the first year of existence. First, the strategy focussed on overutilisation by limiting the number of costly operations such as hysterectomies and elective knee surgeries in developing alternative therapy and treatment. A second route to cut costs was to focus on preventable readmissions by improving case management and discharge planning. Finally, services use of providers outside of the ACO network by patients was to be limited to the greatest extent possible (Blue Shield of California, 2012).

In Germany, the ACO has a strong focus on preventive activities and has developed around 20 preventive and health promotion programmes aimed at patients with specific conditions. It also implemented a series of care management programmes and other measures such as a more rational pharmacotherapy (Hildebrandt et al., 2012). These initiatives appear to have contributed to a reduction in costs. For example, patients treated at participating physicians have lower hospitalisation rates and are more likely to be treated with pharmaceuticals recommended by evidence-based guidelines in the case of heart conditions (Hildebrandt et al., 2012). Data from one of the participating insurers show that two-thirds of the savings among its insured population were realised by lower spending for pharmaceuticals and hospitalisations.

In Spain, remarkable savings have been reported as a result of the application of a new integrated approach to health care delivery focussing on the needs of the patient. Innovations include the attachment of a consultant physician to each health centre as a link to GPs facilitating the implementation of clinical guidelines and effectively reducing the number of inappropriate hospital referrals. Moreover, scope of practice in health centres was enlarged to include onsite X-ray services and accident and emergency departments, and medical care pathways streamlined. Additionally, longer opening hours for outpatient services and elective surgery were established (NHS European Office, 2011). But there are also reports that hospitals managed by Ribera Salud are more selective in their choice of procedures carried out and limit care for patients with chronic conditions, such as for HIV patients (Acerete et al., 2011).

4.6. Conclusion

Recent examples of population-based payments systems show that in some instances provider groups are initially successful in slowing down health spending while maintaining or even improving quality of care and health outcomes. They achieve this by employing resources more efficiently in cutting waste such as double examination and shifting treatment to the most appropriate provider setting. It appears that these innovative modes of payment have at least the potential to enable effective care integration by overcoming care fragmentation. Population-based payments bring together different groups of providers to jointly take responsibility for value-based care centered around the needs of the patient. Making payment dependent on quality is crucial to avoid skimping of care. A welcome side effect of the obligation to report quality measures is that it makes care delivery and performance more transparent. It also is huge step forward towards a more comprehensive and structured data collection on quality with an increased focus on parameters that matter to the patient, such as patient satisfaction and experience as well as outcomes. It remains to be seen whether the positive results can be sustained over a longer time period.

Lessons from ACOs are not easily transferable between health systems

Although health policy objectives that lead to the adoption of population-based payments and ACOs tend to be similar, their actual implementation needs to be analysed in their country-specific context. Health systems differ substantially between OECD countries and it appears that a number of characteristics of a country's health system impact the viability of the different models of the ACOs presented in this chapter.

First, it seems to make a difference whether an ACO is implemented in a country with single or multiple payers. In a regional NHS system like in Spain, care contracts of one health area can only be concluded with regional ministries whereas in the United States, an ACO can have accountable care contracts with Medicare, Medicaid and a number of private insurers whose contents may differ in many aspects (Song and Chokshi, 2015). In the United States, private sector contracts with ACOs generally involve more risk than current Medicare ACO contracts. Moreover, private ACOs have more levers for cost control than Medicare ACOs. They can influence the prices through the negotiation of price discounts whereas prices in the Medicare environment are fixed. Perhaps most importantly, there are significant differences in the population characteristics between private ACOs and Medicare ACOs. Whereas Medicare ACOs are basically limited to the above 65 year old, beneficiaries in private ACOs tend to be younger. This can have important consequences for the care strategy of an ACO as a younger population might be able to benefit more from a wider range of preventive activities aimed at behaviour changes at earlier phases in life. Secondly, there are differences in the legal systems. The ACO model in Germany could not have been implemented if legislation had not been changed to specifically permit public health insurance funds to commission selected health care providers. There are also legal issues related to the question whether payers are able to change the mode of payment to include one- or two-sided risk contracts and whether the emergence of ACOs can be of antitrust concern. In the context of the United States, the question whether the market power of some ACOs can potentially reduce competition and raise prices is under discussion (Shortell et al., 2015). Thirdly, the range of services contracted by ACOs differs between the countries depending on the role of the payer. For example, costs for outpatient pharmaceuticals are not included in benchmark costs for Medicare ACOs and the Alzira model. Long-term care costs are not part of the virtual budget for the German GK. Primary care services were not covered in the first – unsuccessful – Alzira model. The different components included in the benchmark spending will have an impact on the strategy pursued by the ACOs in different countries to reduce total spending.

Can this model be financially sustainable?

The key factor that will decide whether this payment model can gain foothold in a greater number of OECD countries seems to be whether it can be financial sustainable. Although reduced revenues for providers or spending increases for payers might be acceptable in the early years of transition, in the long run, the model needs to be beneficial for all players involved: provider groups, individual providers, payers and patients. Moreover, lessons from the failure of managed care need to be learned. Like some ACOs, Managed Care Organisations also had some initial success in reducing health care spending as they succeeded in negotiating lower prices with health providers who were concerned to lose patients to competitors (Frakt and Mayes, 2012). But after some years of consolidation, health providers were capable of negotiation under more favourable terms pushing health costs back up again.

Payers will continue to support this new population-based payment model if they see reductions in health spending growth and improved quality of care for their insured population and in general get "better value for money". Patients will be in favour if they experience better health care and their financial contributions to the health systems or their health premiums do not increase substantially. The situation for provider groups and individual providers appears to be the most delicate one. For health providers in general, a slowdown in health spending equates with a reduction or limited increase of average revenue. With the possibility of gained savings, provider groups can still financially benefit from this new payment regime. However, this might become complicated in reality if provider groups have shared savings contracts only with a small number of payers (Toussaint et al., 2013). Hence, Medicare encourages ACOs participating in the Pioneer programme to implement shared savings contract with other payers, too. Expanding the

ACO business model is also the aim of the Sacramento ACO which plans to spread into other geographical regions.

While in a number of cases ACOs have succeeded in generating savings in the short run, it is less clear to what the extent this will be feasible in the long run, once the most obvious inefficiencies in an ACO have been addressed. The ability to keep actual costs below the benchmark will largely depend on how savings are defined. In the case where savings are calculated against the benchmark costs of providers outside the ACO programme, a perpetual realisation of annual gains might be a relatively simple task. In the case where costs are benchmarked against projections of the ACO's own historic spending levels, this endeavour might become increasingly difficult with time without compromising quality of care.

ACO managers in the United States believe that the number of patients covered by ACO contracts will grow in the future. Nearly two-third of the leaders of physician-led ACOs believe that they have great potential to improve quality but they are more sceptical about their potential to reduce costs where less than half think ACO contracts can achieve this (Shortell et al., 2015).

Even if the ACO as whole is successful in generating savings and increases its total aggregated revenue, this does not necessarily imply that each individual provider participating in the ACO is benefiting from the payment model. The terms under which savings are used by the ACO and shared among individual providers need to be clear and transparent for all ACO members in order to warrant their full commitment. DeCamp et al. (2014) outline a number of dimensions of fairness to be considered when distributing savings among ACO participants in a "fair and equitable" manner and find that the definition of a unique plan fulfilling this criteria most likely does not exist. It is important to take into account the needs of the individual clinicians as well as organisational and infrastructural needs of the ACO as a whole.

Notes

1. The accountable care contracts in Germany and Spain stipulating population-based payments can be made with legal entities that are non-health providers but may be owned by them. These contractors will also be referred to as ACOs in the remainder of this chapter albeit differences to the Medicare model exist.
2. As discussed in Chapter 3 care groups are contracting partners for health insurers for the implementation of bundled payments for chronic diseases.
3. A risk compensation mechanism exists in the German Statutory Health Insurance Scheme taking into account different distributions of age and diseases of the insured among the 140 public health insurers.
4. This defines the minimum of savings that need to be achieved by an ACO to be eligible to share any savings. Purpose of the risk threshold is to exclude any gains in savings due to random cost variation which cannot be associated to improved efficiency.
5. This defines in monetary terms the value below which savings are shared. This can coincide with the value defined by the minimum savings rate but does not have to.

References

Acerete, B., A. Stafford and P. Stapleton (2011), "Spanish Healthcare Public Private Partnerships: The 'Alzira Model'", *Critical Perspectives on Accounting*, Vol. 22, pp. 533-549.

Addicott, R. and S.M. Shortell (2014), "How Accountable Are Accountable Care Organizations?", *Health Care Management Review*, Vol. 39, No. 4, pp. 270-278.

Alderwick, H., C. Ham and D. Buck (2015), *Population Health Systems. Going Beyond Integrated Care*, The King's Fund, London.

Barnes, A.J. et al. (2014), "Accountable Care Organizations in the USA: Types, Developments and Challenges", *Health Policy*, Vol. 118, pp. 1-7.

Berwick, D.M., T.W. Nolan and J. Whittington (2008), "The Triple Aim: Care, Health and Cost", *Health Affairs*, Vol. 27, No. 3, pp. 759-769.

Blue Shield of California (2012), "Fact Sheet: Blue Shield of California and Accountable Care Organizations (ACOs)", https://www.blueshieldca.com/bsca/documents/about-blue-shield/health-reform/ACO_Blue_Shield_Fact_Sheet_082812.pdf.

Burwell, S.M. (2015), "Setting Value-based Payment Goals – HHS Efforts to improve U.S. Health Care", *New England Journal of Medicine*, Vol. 372, No. 10, pp. 897-899.

Busse, R. and J. Stahl (2014), "Integrated Care Experiences and Outcomes in Germany, the Netherlands, and England", *Health Affairs*, Vol. 33, No. 9, pp. 1549-1558.

Chernew, M.E. et al. (2011), "Private-Payer Innovation in Massachusetts: The 'Alternative Quality Contract'", *Health Affairs*, Vol. 30, No. 1, pp. 51-61.

CMS – Centers for Medicare & Medicaid Services (2015a), "Accountable Care Organisations", http://www.cms.gov/Medicare/Medicare-Fee-for-Service-Payment/ACO/index.html?redirect=/aco/, accessed 30 Sept. 2015.

CMS (2015b), "Medicare Shared Savings Program Shared Savings and Losses and Assignment Methodology", http://www.cms.gov/Medicare/Medicare-Fee-for-Service-Payment/sharedsavingsprogram/Downloads/Shared-Savings-Losses-Assignment-Spec-v2.pdf.

CMS (2015c), "Guide to Quality Performance Scoring Methods for Accountable Care Organizations", http://www.cms.gov/Medicare/Medicare-Fee-for-Service-Payment/sharedsavingsprogram/Downloads/2012-11-ACO-quality-scoring-supplement.pdf.

CMS (2015d), "33 ACO Quality Measures", accessed 30 Sept. 2015, https://www.cms.gov/Medicare/Medicare-Fee-for-Service-Payment/sharedsavingsprogram/Downloads/ACO-Shared-Savings-Program-Quality-Measures.pdf.

CMS (2014), "Medicare ACOs Continue to Succeed in Improving Care, Lowering Cost Growth", Press release 16 Sept. 2014, http://www.cms.gov/Newsroom/MediaReleaseDatabase/Fact-sheets/2014-Fact-sheets-items/2014-09-16.html.

CMS (2013), "Pioneer Accountable Care Organizations Succeed in Improving Care, Lowering Costs", Press release 16 July 2014, http://www.cms.gov/newsroom/mediareleasedatabase/press-releases/2013-press-releases-items/2013-07-16.html.

Colla, C.H. et al. (2014), "First National Survey of ACOs Finds that Physicians Are Playing Strong Leadership and Ownership Roles", *Health Affairs*, Vol. 33, No. 6, pp. 964-971.

Commonwealth Fund (2014), "Hill Physicians Medical Group: A Market-Driven Approach to Accountable Care for Commercially Insured Patients. Case Studies of Accountable Care Systems", The Commonwealth Fund 1770, Vol. 23.

DeCamp, M., J. Sugarman and S. Berkowitz (2014), "Shared Savings in Accountable Care Organisations: How to Determine Fair Distributions", *Journal of the American Medical Association*, Vol. 311, No. 10, pp. 1011-1012.

De Nardi, M. et al. (2015), "Medical Spending of the U.S. Elderly", *NBER Working Paper No. 21270*, Cambridge, United States.

Die Zeit (2015), „Alter schützt vor Fitness nicht", http://www.zeit.de/2015/05/kinzigtal-schwarzwald-gesundheit.

Dupree, J.M. et al. (2014), "Attention to Surgeons and Surgical Care Is Largely Missing from Early Medicare Accountable Care Organizations", *Health Affairs*, Vol. 33, No. 6, pp. 972-979.

Frakt, A.B. and R. Mayes (2012), "Beyond Capitation: How New Payment Experiments Seek to Find the 'Sweet Spot' in Amount of Risk Providers and Payers Bear", *Health Affairs*, Vol. 31, No. 9, pp. 1951-1958.

Gaál, P. et al. (2011), "Hungary: Health System Review", *Health Systems in Transition*, Vol. 13, No. 5, pp. 1-266.

Gesundes Kinzigtal (2014), "Jahresbericht 2013", http://www.gesundes-kinzigtal.de/media/documents/Presse_2014/JB2013_GesundesKinzigtal_Mailversion.pdf.

Hildebrandt, H., T. Schulte and B. Stunder (2012), "Triple Aim in Kinzigtal, Germany", *Journal of Integrated Care*, Vol. 20, No. 4, pp. 205-222.

Kocot, S.L. et al. (2014), "A More Complete Picture of Pioneer ACO Result", Brooking Institute, http://www.brookings.edu/blogs/up-front/posts/2014/10/09-pioneer-aco-results-mcclellan#recent_rr/, accessed 30 Sept. 2015.

Llano, R. (2013), "The Gesundes Kinzigtal Integrated Care Initiative in Germany", *Eurohealth Observer*, Vol. 19,, No. 2, pp. 7-8.

Markovich, P. (2012), "A Global Budget Pilot Project among Provider Partners and Blue Shield of California Led to Savings in First Two Years", *Health Affairs*, Vol. 31, No. 9, pp. 1969-1976.

McClellan, M.B., S.L. Kocot and R. White (2015), "Early Evidence on Medicare ACOs and Next Steps for the Medicare ACO Program (Updated)", *Health Affairs Blog*, 22 January 2015, http://healthaffairs.org/blog/2015/01/22/early-evidence-on-medicare-acos-and-next-steps-for-the-medicare-aco-program/.

McClellan, M. et al. (2014), "Accountable Care around the World: A Framework to Guide Reform Strategies", *Health Affairs*, Vol. 33, No. 9, pp. 1507-1515.

McClellan, M. et al. (2013), "Focusing Accountability on the Outcomes that Matter", Report of the Accountable Care Working Group 2013, World Innovation Summit for Health. Doha.

McWilliams, J.M. et al. (2014), "Changes in Patients' Experiences in Medicare Accountable Care Organizations", *New England Journal of Medicine*, Vol. 371, No. 18, pp. 1715-1724.

Milstein, R. and R. Blankart (2016), "German Case Example", submitted for the OECD Project on Payment Systems, http://www.oecd.org/health/paying-providers.htm.

Mnich, E. et al. (2013), "Outcome Evaluation of a Health Promotion among the Elderly", *Gesundheitswesen*, Vol. 75, No. 02, pp. :e05-e10.

NHS European Office (2011), "The Search for Low-cost Integrated Health Care: The Alzira Model – From the Region of Valencia", The NHS Confederation.

NZ Doctor (2013), "Counties DHB and PHOs Charter New Territory with Alliance Agreement", http://www.nzdoctor.co.nz/news/2013/june-2013/28/counties-dhb-and-phos--charter-new-territory--with-alliance-agreement.aspx.

OECD (2015a), *OECD Reviews of Health Care Quality: Portugal 2015: Raising Standards*, OECD Publishing, Paris, http://dx.doi.org/10.1787/9789264225985-en.

OECD (2015b), "WBG Flagship Study of the Chinese Health System, Delivering person-centred integrated care, Three case studies from OECD Health systems", Paris, OECD, Paris.

RIVM – National Institute for Public Health and the Environment (2014), "Pioneer Sites Move towards Triple Aim", Interim Report, National Population Health Management Monitoring Scheme, RIVM, Bilthoven, December.

Shortell, S.M. et al. (2015), "Accountable Care Organizations: The National Landscape", *Journal of Health Politics, Policy and Law*, Vol. 40, No. 4, pp. 647-668.

Shortell, S.M. et al. (2014a), *Accountable Care Organisations in the United States and England: Testing, Evaluation and Learning What Works*, The King's Fund. London.

Shortell, S.M. et al. (2014b), "A Taxonomy of Accountable Care Organisations for Policy and Practice", *Health Service Research*, Vol. 49, No. 6, pp. 1883-1899.

Song, Z. and D.A. Chokshi (2015), "The Role of Private Payers in Payment Reform", *Journal of the American Medical Association*, Vol. 313, No. 1, pp. 25-26.

Song, Z. et al. (2014), "Changes in Health Spending and Quality 4 Years into Global Payment", *New England Journal of Medicine*, Vol. 371, No. 18, pp. 1704-1714.

Stanton, M.W. and M.K. Rutherford (2005), "The High Concentration of U.S. Health Care Expenditures", *Research in Action No. 19*, Agency for Healthcare Research and Quality, Rockville, United States.

Toussaint, J., A. Milstein and S.M. Shortell (2013), "How the Pioneer ACO Model Needs to Change: Lessons from Its Best-performing ACO", *Journal of the American Medical Association*, Vol. 310, No. 13, pp. 1341-1342.

Weissman, J.S. et al. (2012), "The Design and Application of Shared Savings Programs: Lessons from Early Adopters", *Health Affairs*, Vol. 31, No. 9, pp. 1959-1968.

White House (2014), "Historically Slow Growth in Health Spending Continued in 2013, and Data Show Underlying Slow Cost Growth Is Continuing", http://www.whitehouse.gov/blog/2014/12/03/historically-slow-growth-health-spending-continued-2013-and-data-show-underlying-slo.

ORGANISATION FOR ECONOMIC CO-OPERATION AND DEVELOPMENT

The OECD is a unique forum where governments work together to address the economic, social and environmental challenges of globalisation. The OECD is also at the forefront of efforts to understand and to help governments respond to new developments and concerns, such as corporate governance, the information economy and the challenges of an ageing population. The Organisation provides a setting where governments can compare policy experiences, seek answers to common problems, identify good practice and work to co-ordinate domestic and international policies.

The OECD member countries are: Australia, Austria, Belgium, Canada, Chile, the Czech Republic, Denmark, Estonia, Finland, France, Germany, Greece, Hungary, Iceland, Ireland, Israel, Italy, Japan, Korea, Luxembourg, Mexico, the Netherlands, New Zealand, Norway, Poland, Portugal, the Slovak Republic, Slovenia, Spain, Sweden, Switzerland, Turkey, the United Kingdom and the United States. The European Union takes part in the work of the OECD.

OECD Publishing disseminates widely the results of the Organisation's statistics gathering and research on economic, social and environmental issues, as well as the conventions, guidelines and standards agreed by its members.

OECD PUBLISHING, 2, rue André-Pascal, 75775 PARIS CEDEX 16
(81 2016 09 1 P) ISBN 978-92-64-25820-4 – 2016

www.ingramcontent.com/pod-product-compliance
Ingram Content Group UK Ltd.
Pitfield, Milton Keynes, MK11 3LW, UK
UKHW051503290926
15471UKWH00008B/1376

9 789264 258204